Self-Assessment
by Ten Teachers

Self-Assessment by Ten Teachers

EMQs, MCQs, SAQs and OSCEs in Obstetrics and Gynaecology

Jeremy C Brockelsby BSc MB BS PhD MRCOG
Consultant in Obstetrics and Feto Maternal Medicine
at The Rosie Maternity Hospital, Addenbrookes Hospital,
Cambridge University Hospital NHS Foundation Trust, Cambridge, UK

Christian Phillips BSc (Hons) BM DM MRCOG
Consultant Gynaecologist, Basingstoke and
North Hampshire NHS Foundation Trust,
Basingstoke, Hampshire, UK

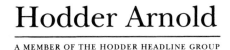

Hodder Arnold

A MEMBER OF THE HODDER HEADLINE GROUP

First published in Great Britain in 2007 by
Hodder Arnold, an imprint of Hodder Education and a member of the Hodder Headline Group,
338 Euston Road, London NW1 3BH

http://www.hoddereducation.co.uk

Figures 8.1–8.10, 8.12 and 8.14–8.16 reproduced and adapted from Monga A (ed) *Gynaecology By Ten Teachers*, 18th edition (London: Edward Arnold 2006) were also from Campbell S and Monga A (eds), *Gynaecology By Ten Teachers*, 17th edition (London: Edward Arnold 2000).

Figure 4.1, adapted from Baker PN (ed) *Obstetrics By Ten Teachers*, 18th edition (London: Edward Arnold 2006) was also from Campbell S and Lees C (eds), *Obstetrics By Ten Teachers*, 17th edition (London: Edward Arnold 2000).

Whilst the advice and information in this book are believed to be true and accurate at the date of going to press, neither the authors nor the publisher can accept any legal responsibility or liability for any errors or omissions that may be made. In particular, (but without limiting the generality of the preceding disclaimer) every effort has been made to check drug dosages; however it is still possible that errors have been missed. Furthermore, dosage schedules are constantly being revised and new side-effects recognized. For these reasons the reader is strongly urged to consult the drug companies' printed instructions before administering any of the drugs recommended in this book.

British Library Cataloguing in Publication Data
A catalogue record for this book is available from the British Library

Library of Congress Cataloging-in-Publication Data
A catalog record for this book is available from the Library of Congress

ISBN   978-0-340-90615-6
ISBN [ISE]   978-0-340-94691-6 (International Students' Edition, restricted territorial availability)

1 2 3 4 5 6 7 8 9 10

Commissioning Editor: Sara Purdy
Project Editor: Jane Tod
Production Controller: Lindsay Smith
Cover Design: Nichola Smith
Indexer: Indexing Specialists (UK) Ltd

Typeset in 9.25/12 Minion by Charon Tec Ltd (A Macmillan Company), Chennai, India
www.charontec.com
Printed and bound in Malta

What do you think about this book? Or any other Hodder Arnold title?
Please visit our website: www.hoddereducation.co.uk

Contents

I dedicate this book to my father, Tommy Brockelsby, who passed away during the completion of this book; and to my wife Clare Brockelsby, who put up with all the hours I spent away from the family while writing.

Jeremy Brockelsby

To Tanja, Jonny and Tilly

Christian Phillips

Acknowledgements

Self-Assessment by Ten Teachers is indebted to *Gynaecology by Ten Teachers* and *Obstetrics by Ten Teachers*. In particular, Jeremy Brockelsby, Christian Phillips and the publishers would like to thank Philip N Baker, editor of the 18th edition of the obstetrics volume, and Ash Monga, editor of the 18th edition of the gynaecology volume, and the contributors to both these volumes who collectively have supported the concept and have kindly allowed for their material to be the basis for this student revision guide:

Keith Edmonds · David W Purdie · Griffith Jones · Catherine Nelson-Piercy
Ailsa E Gebbie · Fran Reader · Lucy Kean · Janet Rennie
Phillip Hay · W. Patrick Soutter · Louise Kenny · Abdul Sultan
Susan Ingamells · R. W. Stones · Gary Mires · Phillip Hay
Jane Norman · Ian Johnson · Alec McEwan

In addition, the authors and the publishers would also like to extend their thanks to the editors of and contributors to the 17th editions of *Gynaecology by Ten Teachers* and *Obstetrics by Ten Teachers* who have not been actively involved in the preparation of this self-assessment volume, but whose input in these earlier editions led to the introduction of many of the concepts and features reflected here:

Stuart Campbell, James Drife, William Dunlop, D Keith Edmonds, Ailsa E Gebbie, Jason Gardosi, Donald Gibb, JG Grudzinskas, Kevin Harrington, Phillip E Hay, Des Holden, Eric Janiaux, Richard Johanson, Simon M Kelly, Christoph Lees, Ash Monga, Geeta Nargund, Kypros Nicolaides, Jane E Norman, Margaret R Oates, PM Sean O'Brien, David W Purdie, Fran Reader, Michael Robson, Neil Sebire, Robert W Shaw, W Patrick Soutter, R William Stones, E Malcolm Symonds, Basky Thilaganathan, J Guy Thorpe-Beeston.

Commonly used abbreviations

ACTH	adrenocorticotrophic hormone
AIDS	acquired immunodeficiency syndrome
AP	anterior–posterior
BMI	body mass index
BP	blood pressure
BSO	bilateral salpingo-oophorectomy
BV	bacterial vaginosis
CAH	congenital adrenal hyperplasia
CEMACH	Confidential Enquiry into Maternal and Child Health
CESDI	Confidential Enquiry into Stillbirths and Deaths in Infancy
CGIN	cervical glandular intraepithelial neoplasia
CIN	cervical intraepithelial neoplasia
CMV	cytomegalovirus
COCP	combined oral contraceptive pill
CPD	cephalopelvic disproportion
CRF	corticotrophin-releasing factor
CT	computerized tomography
CTG	cardiotocography
CVS	chorionic villus sampling
DFA	direct fluorescent antibody
DVT	deep vein thrombosis
E2	oestradiol
ECV	external cephalic version
EDD	expected date of delivery
ELISA	enzyme-linked immunosorbent assay
ERPC	evacuation of retained products of conception
FBC	full blood count
FSH	follicle-stimulating hormone
FTA	fluorescent treponemal antibody
GFR	glomerular filtration rate
GnRH	gonadotrophin-releasing hormone
GP	general practitioner
Hb	haemoglobin
hCG	human chorionic gonadotrophin
HDL	high-density lipoprotein
HIV	human immunodeficiency virus
HPV	human papilloma virus
HRT	hormone replacement therapy
HSV	high vaginal swab
IGF	insulin-like growth factor
IHC	intrahepatic cholestasis
IUCD	intrauterine contraceptive device
IUD	intrauterine device
IUGR	intrauterine growth restriction
IUS	intrauterine system
IVF	*in-vitro* fertilization
IVP	intravenous pyelogram
LDL	low-density lipoprotein
LFT	liver function test
LH	luteinizing hormone
LLETZ	large loop excision of the transformation zone
LMP	last menstrual period
LNG-IUS	levonorgestrel intrauterine system
MCV	mean corpuscular volume
MSSU	mid-stream specimen of urine
NHS	National Health Service
NSAID	non-steroidal anti-inflammatory drug
NTD	neural tube defect
P4	progesterone
PCOS	polycystic ovarian syndrome
PE	pulmonary embolus/embolism
PID	pelvic inflammatory disease
PROM	preterm rupture of the membranes
RCOG	Royal College of Obstetricians and Gynaecologists
RMI	relative malignancy index
sβhCG	serum β-human chorionic gonadotrophin
SSRIs	selective serotonin reuptake inhibitors
TAH	total abdominal hysterectomy
TCRE	transcervical resection of endometrium
TDF	testicular development factor
TFT	thyroid function test
TPHA	*Treponema pallidum* haemagglutination assay
TPPA	*Treponema pallidum* particle agglutination
TSH	thyroid-stimulating hormone
TVT	tension-free vaginal tape
USI	urodynamic stress incontinence
VDRL	Venereal Disease Research Laboratories
VTE	venous thromboembolism

Obstetrics

Extended matching questions

1 Maternal and perinatal mortality: the confidential enquiry

A Maternal death
B Direct maternal death
C Indirect maternal death
D Maternal mortality rate
E Perinatal death
F Perinatal mortality rate
G Stillbirth
H None of the above

For each description below, choose the SINGLE most appropriate answer from the above list of options. Each option may be used once, more than once, or not at all.

1 Death of a woman while pregnant, or within 42 days of termination of pregnancy, from any cause related to, or aggravated by, the pregnancy or its management, but not from accidental or incidental death.
2 The number of stillbirths and early neonatal deaths per 1000 live births and stillbirths.
3 Fetal death occurring between 20 + 0 weeks and 23 + 6 weeks. If the gestation is not certain all births of at least 300 g are reported.
4 Death resulting from previous existing disease, or disease that developed during pregnancy and which was not due to direct obstetric cause, but which was aggravated by the effects of pregnancy that are due to direct or indirect maternal causes.

2 Conception, implantation and embryology

A Paramesonephric ducts
B Mesonephric ducts
C Primitive streak

D Anterior neuropore
E Posterior neuropore
F Mesoderm

G Ectoderm
H Endoderm

For each description below, choose the SINGLE most appropriate answer from the above list of options. Each option may be used once, more than once, or not at all.

1 The structure that give rise to the uterus.
2 The structure that give rise to the somites.
3 The structure that gives rise to the gastrointestinal tract.
4 The structure that defines caudal and cephalic poles.

3 Physiological changes in pregnancy: uterus and cervix

A Inhibin

B Progesterone

C Oestradiol

D Insulin-like growth factors I and II
E Human chorionic gonadotrophin
F Human placental lactogen

G Corticotrophin-releasing factor

H None of the above

For each description below, choose the SINGLE most appropriate answer from the above list of options. Each option may be used once, more than once, or not at all.

1 A peptide that is used within the triple test.
2 A substance that is produced by trophoblast from mid-pregnancy.
3 A peptide hormone produced within the myometrium.
4 A pregnancy-specific hormone that has thyrotrophic activity.

4 Normal fetal development: the fetal heart

A The ductus venous
B The ductus arteriosus
C Foramen ovale
D Left atrium

E Right atrium
F Mitral valve
G Tricuspid valve
H Umbilical vein

I Umbilical artery
J Intra-atrial septum
K Intraventricular septum
L None of the above

For each description below, choose the SINGLE most appropriate answer from the above list of options. Each option may be used once, more than once, or not at all.

1 Location of the patent foramen ovale.
2 Vessel that carries oxygenated blood from the placenta and, in adult life, forms part of the falciform ligament.
3 Blood from the inferior and superior vena cava is directed across this structure in neonatal life.
4 Vessel that shunts blood away from the liver.

5 Antenatal care

A Triple test	**E** Dating scan	**I** Biophysical scan
B Ferritin	**F** Syphilis	**J** Anatomy scan
C Mid-stream specimen of urine (MSSU)	**G** Protein dip stix	**K** Nuchal translucency scan
D Full blood count (FBC)	**H** Urate	

For each description below, choose the SINGLE most appropriate answer from the above list of options. Each option may be used once, more than once, or not at all.

1 A second trimester test for Down's syndrome.
2 A fetal viability test.
3 A screening test for pre-eclampsia.

6 Antenatal imaging and fetal assessment

A Variable decelerations	**E** Fetal heart rate accelerations	**I** Biophysical profile
B Late decelerations	**F** Antenatal Doppler	**J** None of the above
C Early decelerations	**G** Doppler in labour	
D Baseline variability	**H** Diagnostic ultrasound	

For each description below, choose the SINGLE most appropriate answer from the above list of options. Each option may be used once, more than once, or not at all.

1 Reflection of the normal fetal autonomic nervous system.
2 Assessment of fetal breathing, gross body movements, fetal tone, reactive fetal heart rate and amniotic fluid.
3 Transient reduction in the fetal heart rate of 15 beats per minute or more, lasting for more than 15 seconds.
4 Transient increase in the fetal heart rate of 15 beats per minute or more, lasting for more than 15 seconds.

7 Prenatal diagnosis

A Spina bifida	**D** Thalassemia	**G** Turner's syndrome
B Down's syndrome	**E** Cerebral palsy	**H** Fragile X
C Duchenne muscular dystrophy	**F** Klinefelter's syndrome	**I** None of the above

For each description below, choose the SINGLE most appropriate answer from the above list of options. Each option may be used once, more than once, or not at all.

1 The diagnosis may be suspected on ultrasound by the observation of the lemon and banana signs.
2 Measurement of the maternal serum hormones during the second trimester offers an effective screening modality.
3 Prenatal diagnosis is available by the demonstration of multiple repeats (>200) in a male fetus.
4 Affected individuals are infertile males with a slightly reduced intelligence, testicular dysgenesis and a tall stature.

8 Second trimester miscarriage

A	Threatened miscarriage	**D**	Septic miscarriage	**G**	Urinary tract infection
B	Inevitable miscarriage	**E**	Incompetent cervix	**H**	None of the above
C	Missed miscarriage	**F**	Chorioamnionitis		

For each description below, choose the SINGLE most appropriate answer from the above list of options. Each option may be used once, more than once, or not at all.

1 A 23-year-old woman presents at 13 weeks of amenorrhea. She is complaining of low backache and suprapubic discomfort. Routine examination of the patient's abdomen reveals that there is suprapubic tenderness. Examination of her vital signs reveals pyrexia of 37.7°C and a tachycardia of 90 beats per minute. Internal examination reveals that the cervix is closed. Urine dipstix demonstrates leucocytes and nitrites.

2 A 23-year-old woman presents at 20 weeks of amenorrhea in her second pregnancy. The first pregnancy had unfortunately ended at 19 weeks with a miscarriage after premature rupture of the fetal membranes. She is complaining of low backache, feeling warm and a slight vaginal loss. She has pyrexia of 38°C and a pulse of 98 beats per minute. Routine examination of the patient's abdomen reveals that there is tenderness suprapubically. Speculum examination reveals a slightly open cervix and fluid draining.

3 A 23-year-old woman presents at 13 weeks of amenorrhea. She is complaining of vaginal bleeding, low backache and suprapubic discomfort. Routine examination of the patient's abdomen reveals that there is suprapubic tenderness. Examination of her vital signs demonstrates that she is apyrexial. Internal examination reveals that the cervix is closed. Urine dipstix is unremarkable.

4 A 32-year-old woman presents in her first pregnancy at 20 weeks of amenorrhea. She is complaining of minor discomfort in the lower abdomen. Her pulse and blood pressure are within the normal range and she is apyrexial. Abdominal examination is unremarkable. However, speculum examination reveals a slightly open cervix. A transvaginal ultrasound scan demonstrates the cervical canal to be 2 cm long and funnelling of the membranes is present.

9 Antenatal obstetric complications

Antepartum haemorrhage

A	Placenta praevia	**D**	Threatened miscarriage	**G**	Vasa praevia
B	Placenta abruption	**E**	Ectopic pregnancy	**H**	Vaginal infection
C	Complete miscarriage	**F**	Cancer of the cervix	**I**	None of the above

For each description below, choose the SINGLE most appropriate answer from the above list of options. Each option may be used once, more than once, or not at all.

1 A 32-year-old woman presented to the delivery suite. She was 28 weeks pregnant in her second pregnancy. An ultrasound scan at 12 weeks had confirmed a twin pregnancy. She was admitted complaining of bleeding per vaginum; this was bright red in nature and painless.

2 A 34-year-old woman presents to casualty. She has a history of pelvic inflammatory disease. She is 7 weeks pregnant by her dates. She is complaining of left-side abdominal pain and brown discharge. On examination, she is tender in the left iliac fossa and the cervix is closed.

3 A 26-year-old woman presents to casualty. She has a history of pelvic inflammatory disease. She is 7 weeks pregnant by her dates and is complaining of bright red bleeding per vaginum. She also complains of suprapubic tenderness. On examination, there is blood in the vagina and the cervix is closed.

4 A 32-year-old woman presented to the delivery suite. She was 34 weeks pregnant in her first pregnancy. She was admitted complaining of severe abdominal pain, and bright red bleeding and clots per vaginum. On examination, the uterus was painful and there were palpable contractions.

10 Twins and higher order multiple gestations

A Miscarriage
B Diachorionic diamniotic twins
C Monochorionic monoamniotic twins
D Twin–twin transfusion syndrome

E Preterm labour
F Nuchal translucency
G Triple test
H Monochorionic diamniotic twins

I Pre-eclampsia
J Monozygotic twins
K None of the above

For each description below, choose the SINGLE most appropriate answer from the above list of options. Each option may be used once, more than once, or not at all.

1 The observation of the lambda sign on an early pregnancy scan confirms the diagnosis.
2 Death or handicap of the co-twin occurs in 25 per cent of cases.
3 The chance that at least one of the twin pair is affected by a chromosomal defect is twice as high as for a singleton pregnancy.
4 Placental vascular anastomoses allow communication between the two feto-placental circulations. In some twin pregnancies, imbalance in the blood flow across these arteriovenous communications occurs.

11 Disorders of placentation

The clinical management of hypertension in pregnancy

A Magnesium hydroxide
B Oral antihypertensive
C Oral diuretic
D Monitor blood pressure.
E Renal function tests

F 24-hour urinary protein
G Admission for observation and investigation.
H Fetal ultrasound

I Immediate Caesarean section
J Induction of labour
K Intravenous antihypertensive
L None of the above

For each description below, choose the SINGLE most appropriate action from the above list of options. Each option may be used once, more than once, or not at all.

1 At 34 weeks, a 80 kg woman complains of persistent headaches and 'flashing lights'. There is no hyper-reflexia and her blood pressure (BP) is 155/100 mmHg.
2 At 33 weeks, a 31-year-old primigravida is found to have BP of 145/95 mmHg. At her first visit at 12 weeks, the BP was 145/85 mmHg. She has no proteinuria but she is found to have oedema to her knees.
3 A 29-year-old woman has an uneventful first pregnancy to 31 weeks. She is then admitted as an emergency with epigastric pain. During the first 3 hours, her BP rises from 150/100 to 170/119 mmHg. A dipstick test reveals she has 3+ proteinuria. The fetal cardiotocogram is normal.
4 A 32-year-old woman in her second pregnancy presents to her general practitioner (GP) at 12 weeks' gestation. She was mildly hypertensive in both of her previous pregnancies. Her BP is 150/100 mmHg. Two weeks later, at the hospital antenatal clinic, her BP is 155/100 mmHg.

12 Medical diseases of pregnancy

Drugs used in pregnancy

A Calcium supplements
B Erythromycin
C Nifedipine

D Ritodrine
E Ursodeoxycholic acid
F Magnesium sulphate

G Oral labetolol
H Ferrous sulphate
I None of the above

For each description below, choose the SINGLE most appropriate drug treatment from the above list of options. Each option may be used once, more than once, or not at all.

1 A 27-year-old woman presents at 33 weeks in her first pregnancy. She is complaining of generalized itching, worse on the palms of her hands and soles of her feet. Abdominal examination is unremarkable. Blood investigations reveal that she has increased bile acids.
2 A 23-year-old primigravid women presents at 31 weeks. At her 12 weeks booking visit she was normotensive and had no history of epilepsy. She is admitted as an emergency having had a seizure. On admission, her blood pressure is 150/110 mmHg and dipstick urine analysis reveals 3+ proteinuria.
3 A 32-year-old woman presents in her second pregnancy at 29 weeks. Her first pregnancy had been uncomplicated, however, she had delivered at 36 weeks' gestation. She is admitted with a history of sudden gush of fluid per vaginum. On examination her abdomen is consistent with a 29-week pregnancy. Speculum examination reveals copious amounts of clear fluid. Temperature and pulse are normal.
4 A 25-year-old Asian woman in her third pregnancy presents to clinic at 24 weeks of her pregnancy. She is complaining of tiredness and lethargy. Abdominal examination is unremarkable. Dipstix urine analysis demonstrates 3+ glycosuria. A full blood count reveals haemoglobin of 11 g/dL. An oral glucose tolerance test shows a fasting blood glucose of 8.1 mmol/L.

13 Perinatal infections

A Toxoplasmosis
B Cytomegalovirus
C *Varicella zoster*
D Cocksackie B virus

E *Listeria monocytogenes*
F *Herpes simplex*
G *Chlamydia trachomatis*

H Gonorrhoea
I Trichmoniasis
J None of the above

For each description below, choose the SINGLE most appropriate answer from the above list of options. Each option may be used once, more than once, or not at all.

1 A bacterium that is found in sewage, but can grow in refrigerated food, including meat, eggs, and dairy products.
2 A protozoan parasite that may be acquired from exposure to cat faeces or from eating uncooked meats.
3 In children it causes a viral exanthema know as 'fifth disease'.
4 Primary infection usually presents within 7 days of exposure and may be accompanied by wide lesions around the vulva, vagina, and cervix.

14 Labour

Mechanism of labour

A Descent	**D** Flexion	**G** Internal rotation
B Extension	**E** External rotation	**H** None of the above
C Engagement	**F** Restitution	

For each description below, choose the SINGLE most appropriate answer from the above list of options. Each option may be used once, more than once, or not at all.

1 After the head delivers through the vulva, it immediately aligns with the fetal shoulders.
2 The occiput escapes from underneath the symphysis pubis, which acts as fulcrum.
3 The anterior shoulder lies inferior to the symphysis pubis and delivers first, and the posterior shoulder delivers subsequently.
4 When the widest part of the presenting part has passed successfully through the pelvic inlet.

15 Obstetric emergencies

Collapse

A Simple faint	**D** Pulmonary embolism	**G** Hypoglycaemia
B Epileptic fit	**E** Eclampsia	**H** Ectopic pregnancy
C Subarachnoid haemorrhage	**F** Haemorrhage	**I** None of the above

For each description below, choose the SINGLE most appropriate diagnosis from the above list of options. Each option may be used once, more than once, or not at all.

1 A 37-year-old woman in her second pregnancy has delivered a live male infant. She has no past medical history of note. Ten minutes after delivery, she complains of a sudden onset severe occipital headache that is associated with vomiting. Shortly after this, she losses consciousness and is unresponsive to any stimuli.
2 A 23-year-old woman who is 32 weeks pregnant presents to delivery suite. She complains of feeling generally unwell. Clinical examination reveals a 28-week size fetus. Her blood pressure was noted to be 120/90 mmHg and on urine analysis 2+ protein was present. During the clinical examination, she has a seizure.
3 A 32-year-old woman who has had an emergency Caesarean section is on the postnatal ward. She suddenly becomes breathless and complains of central chest pain. She subsequently loses consciousness.

16 The puerperium

Postpartum pyrexia

A	Pylelophritis	E	Meningitis	I	Breast abscess
B	Mastitis	F	Endometritis	J	Chest infection
C	Pneumonia	G	Wound infection	K	None of the above
D	Deep vein thrombosis	H	Retained products of conception		

For each description below, choose the SINGLE most appropriate answer from the above list of options. Each option may be used once, more than once, or not at all.

1 A 30-year-old woman is admitted from home. She had an uncomplicated pregnancy and a normal vaginal delivery 4 days previously. She presented with feeling generally unwell associated with heavy, fresh, vaginal bleeding and clots. On examination, she has a temperature of 38.3°C. Abdominal examination reveals mild suprapubic tenderness. Vaginal examination revealed blood clots and the cervix admits a finger and is enlarged and bulky.

2 A 26-year-old woman is admitted 7 days after having a Caesarean section, which was performed for failure to progress after augmentation for prolonged rupture of the fetal membranes. She is generally unwell and complains of a foul-smelling vaginal discharge. On examination, she has a temperature of 39.0°C. Abdominal examination reveals suprapubic tenderness. Vaginal examination confirms the offensive discharge and uterine tenderness.

3 A 32-year-old woman is seen 3 days after having a Caesarean section. The Caesarean section was performed as an emergency for placental abruption and was carried out under general anaesthesia. She is complaining that she is generally unwell and has been coughing up green sputum. On examination, she has a temperature of 38.0°C and a pulse of 90 beats per minute. The respiratory rate is 30 inspirations per minute and she using her accessory respiratory muscles. Abdominal and pelvic examinations are unremarkable. Chest examination reveals purulent sputum and coarse crackles of auscultation.

17 Psychiatric disorders in pregnancy and the puerperium

A	Baby blues	D	Schizophrenia	G	Depression
B	Postnatal depression	E	Puerperal psychosis	H	None of the above
C	Panic disorders	F	Bipolar affective disorder		

For each description below, choose the SINGLE most appropriate answer from the above list of options. Each option may be used once, more than once, or not at all.

1 A 40-year-old woman presents on the fifth day after a normal delivery. Her husband has brought her in to accident and emergency, after he noticed an abrupt change in her behaviour. He describes her as confused, restless and is expressing thoughts of self-harm.

2 A 23-year-old woman, who had a normal delivery 12 hours earlier, is noted by the ward staff to be having difficulties sleeping, is overactive and expresses feelings of excitement.

3 A 23-year-old woman presents at a booking clinic. She is 7 weeks pregnant in her first pregnancy and has been referred by the community midwife for consultant care. She is taking lithium and carbamazepine.

4 A 32-year-old woman who had an emergency Caesarean section 2 days earlier, is noted by the midwives on the ward to be having sleeping difficulties, and is tearful and short tempered.

18 Neonatology

A Erythema toxicum	**E** Subgaleal haemorrhage	**I** Milia
B Erb's palsy	**F** Transient tachypnoea of the newborn	**J** Port wine stain
C Klumpke's palsy	**G** Respiratory distress syndrome	**K** None of the above
D Necrotizing entrocolitis	**H** Cerebral palsy	

For each description below, choose the SINGLE most appropriate answer from the above list of options. Each option may be used once, more than once, or not at all.

1 A newborn baby of 36 weeks' gestation, present with cyanosis, tachypnoea, grunting and recession.
2 In a newborn postnatal check of a term baby delivered by vaginal breech, the attending senior house officer notes that there is a claw hand with inability to extend the fingers.
3 The senior house officer is asked by the midwives to review a 3-day-old baby. The baby has an oval erythematous rash with white pinpoint heads.

EMQ answers

1 Maternal and perinatal mortality: the confidential enquiry

1 A   **2** F   **3** H   **4** C

Fetal death occurring between 20 + 0 weeks and 23 + 6 completed weeks. If the gestation is not sure, all births of at least 300 g are reported. This is the definition of a late fetal loss and, as such, does not fit with any of the answers given above.

See Chapter 3, *Obstetrics by Ten Teachers*, 18th edition.

2 Conception, implantation and embryology

1 A   **2** F   **3** H   **4** C

The pararmesonephric or Mullerian ducts develop into the uterus, uterine cervix and the fallopian tubes along with the upper third of the vagina. The somites are a series of mesoderm tissue blocks that are found on each side of the neural tube. The gastrointestinal tract is the main organ system derived from endodermal layer. The primitive streak determines symmetry and defines the caudal and cephalic poles of the embryo.

See Chapter 4, *Obstetrics by Ten Teachers*, 18th edition.

3 Physiological changes in pregnancy: uterus and cervix

1 E   **2** G   **3** D   **4** E

Human chrionic gonadotrophin (hCG) is the peptide that is incorporated into triple test. The alpha-subunit of hCG differs only slightly from the alpha-subunits of luteinizing hormone (LH), follicle-stimulating hormone (FSH) and thyroid-stimulating hormone (TSH), and can interact with these receptors. Insulin and insulin-like growth factors (IGFs) are important for fetal growth. Both IGF-I and II are produced within the uterus. From mid-pregnancy, the trophoblast is capable of producing corticotrophin-releasing factor (CRF) and this stimulates the fetal pituitary to increase fetal adrenocorticotrophic hormone.

See Chapter 5, *Obstetrics by Ten Teachers*, 18th edition.

4 Normal fetal development: the fetal heart

1 J   **2** H   **3** G   **4** A

The foramen ovale shunts blood from the right to the left atrium. With the closure of the foremen ovale at birth, blood drains from the inferior and superior vena cava into the right atrium and is directed across the tricuspid value into the right ventricle.

See Chapter 6, *Obstetrics by Ten Teachers*, 18th edition.

5 Antenatal care

1 A   **2** E   **3** G

The triple test is a biochemical-screening test for Down's syndrome. The dating scan has several specific aims, which include fetal viability, dating, diagnosis and chorionicity of twins. Quantification of protein in combination with blood pressure determination is the main screening test for pre-eclampsia.

See Chapter 7, *Obstetrics by Ten Teachers*, 18th edition.

6 Antenatal imaging and fetal assessment

1 D   2 I   3 J   4 E

Although variable, early and late decelerations all have a component in their definition that describes transient reductions in the fetal heart rate of 15 beats per minute or more, lasting for more than 15 seconds, their definitions require information as to whether the deceleration occurs with or after a contraction. A transient increase in the fetal heart rate of 15 beats per minute or more, lasting for more than 15 seconds, is the definition of fetal heart rate acceleration. It requires no timing with a contraction for its definition.

See Chapter 8, *Obstetrics by Ten Teachers*, 18th edition.

7 Prenatal diagnosis

1 A   2 B   3 H   4 F

The most common presenting signs of spina bifida on ultrasound examination are the lemon-shaped skulls and the banana-shaped cerebellum.

See Chapter 9, *Obstetrics by Ten Teachers*, 18th edition.

8 Second trimester miscarriage

1 G   2 F   3 A   4 E

Abdominal discomfort and suprapubic pain are common symptoms that present to obstetricians. However, the pyrexia and leucocytes within the urine would suggest that this is a urinary tract infection, which should be treated with antibiotics. The presentation of ruptured membranes and pyrexia would suggest chorionamnionitis, which should be treated with high-dose antibiotics and possibly termination of the pregnancy for maternal health. The ultrasound examination that demonstrated cervical dilatation and funnelling is suggestive of an incompetent cervix. This could be treated by the insertion of a cervical cerclarage.

See Chapter 10, *Obstetrics by Ten Teachers*, 18th edition.

9 Antenatal obstetric complications

1 A   2 E   3 D   4 B

The most likely diagnosis for a twin pregnancy presenting with painless vaginal bleeding is a placenta praevia. The twin pregnancy increases the surface area of the placenta and, therefore, increases the chances of it being low within the uterine cavity. The most likely diagnosis for a woman with a previous history of pelvic inflammatory disease and iliac fossa pain is an ectopic pregnancy. Although pelvic inflammatory disease is associated with Fallopian tube damage and increased risk of tubal pregnancy, it does not occur in all women with ectopic pregnancy. Therefore, it may be in the history of a woman with a threatened miscarriage.

See Chapter 11, *Obstetrics by Ten Teachers*, 18th edition.

10 Twins and higher order multiple gestations

1 B   2 J   3 K   4 D

The chance that at least one of a diazygotic twin pair being affected by a chromosomal defect is twice as high as for a singleton pregnancy. It should be noted that at least 10 per cent of diachorionic diamniotic twins develop from a single zygote and, therefore, have a risk of Down's syndrome based on maternal age only.

See Chapter 12, *Obstetrics by Ten Teachers*, 18th edition.

11 Disorders of placentation

1 G   **2** D   **3** K   **4** B

At 34 weeks' gestation, the mostly likely diagnosis is pre-eclampsia. However, the diagnosis of pre-eclampsia requires urinary protein quantification. Therefore, the management would be for admission and further investigation. A 31-year-old woman with a booking blood pressure of 145/85 mmHg has chronic hypertension. During pregnancy, the blood pressure initially falls and then rises in the third trimester; therefore, this may be a normal physiological response for this woman and, as such, the blood pressure should be monitored. A blood pressure ranging from 150/100 to 170/119 mmHg with significant proteinuria indicates pre-eclampsia. A woman with a blood pressure within this range needs treatment with intravenous antihypertensives.

See Chapters 13 and 15, *Obstetrics by Ten Teachers*, 18th edition.

12 Medical diseases of pregnancy

1 E   **2** F   **3** B   **4** I

Ursodeoxycholic acid is used in the symptomatic treatment of obstetric cholestasis. It chelates bile acids and reduces the itching associated with the disorder. Magnesium sulphate has been shown to reduce the chances of a patient having a further seizure related to pre-eclampsia. A woman presenting with tiredness, glycosuria and a fasting blood glucose of 8.1 mmol/L has diabetes and may require insulin to control blood glucose.

See Chapter 15, *Obstetrics by Ten Teachers*, 18th edition.

13 Perinatal infections

1 E   **2** A   **3** I   **4** F

Listeria monocytogenes is a Gram-positive rod. It is an important cause of a wide spectrum of human diseases. Toxoplasmosis is a protozoan that can produce congenital or postnatal infections in humans. Congenital infections occur when non-immune mothers are infected with the protozoan and are of greater severity. Fifths disease is caused by parvovirus B19.

See Chapter 16, *Obstetrics by Ten Teachers*, 18th edition.

14 Labour

1 F   **2** B   **3** H   **4** C

The mechanism of labour refers to the series of changes that occur in the position and attitude of the fetus during its passage through the birth canal. The process involves engagement, descent, flexion, internal rotation, extension, restitution, external rotation, and delivery of the shoulders and fetal body. Engagement is side to have occurred when the widest part of the presenting part has passed successfully through the inlet.

See Chapter 17, *Obstetrics by Ten Teachers*, 18th edition.

15 Obstetric emergencies

1 C   2 E   3 D

The history of a sudden onset of occipital headaches with associated vomiting should raise the suspicion of sub-arachnoid haemorrhage. The associated loss of consciousness would point to the diagnosis of subarachnoid haemorrhage. Although migraine and hypercalcaemia could present with this history, they are not options available. The definitive diagnosis would be confirmed with brain imaging. The combination of hypertension and proteinuria combined with a collapse would be eclampsia until proven otherwise.

See Chapter 19, *Obstetrics by Ten Teachers*, 18th edition.

16 The puerperium

1 G   2 F   3 C

The most likely diagnosis of an enlarged uterus and associated temperature is retained products of conception. She initially needs blood cultures and intravenous antibiotics. This should be followed by a surgical evacuation of the uterus. The differential diagnosis for a woman who presents after a Caesarean section with a temperature and abdominal pain is a wound infection, uterine infection or urinary tract infection. Caesarean section increases the risk of uterine infection and this is confirmed by the presence of an offensive discharge. This is unlikely to be retained products, as the uterine cavity is checked manually after a Caesarean section. A urinary tract infection would have dysuria and urine analysis would be abnormal. The differential diagnosis of a woman who presents with a temperature and chest signs is a chest infection, pneumonia or pulmonary embolism. The most likely diagnosis with purulent sputum is pneumonia, which should be treated with antibiotics.

See Chapter 20, *Obstetrics by Ten Teachers*, 18th edition.

17 Psychiatric disorders in pregnancy and the puerperium

1 E   2 F   3 H   4 A

Puerperal psychosis affects approximately 1 in 1000 women. It presents rarely before the third postpartum day, but usually does so before 4 weeks. The onset is characteristically abrupt, with rapidly changing clinical picture. The patient should be referred urgently to a psychiatrist and will require admission to a psychiatric unit. It is common for women in the first 24–48 hours to experience an elevation in mood, a feeling of excitement and some overactivity. This is termed to the postnatal 'pinks'. Bipolar affective disorder is usually controlled with a combination of mood-stabilizing drugs (lithium), antidepressants and neuroleptics. Lithium carries a risk of causing cardiac defects if used in the first trimester.

See Chapter 21, *Obstetrics by Ten Teachers*, 18th edition.

18 Neonatology

1 G   2 C   3 A

Damage to the lowest roots of the brachial plexus (C8 and T1) is unusual but includes Klumpke's palsy due to birth during breech delivery where the arm remains above the head.

See Chapter 22, *Obstetrics by Ten Teachers*, 18th edition.

Chapter 2

Multiple choice questions

History and examination

1   **With regard to the obstetric history:**
a) Pregnancy is dated from conception.
b) Parity is the total number of pregnancies regardless of how they ended.
c) It is recommended that women should be seen on their own at least once.
d) A family history of pre-eclampsia should trigger increased antenatal surveillance.
e) The last menstrual period is reliable if the cycles are irregular.

2   **The following terms are appropriate:**
a) Lie: cephalic.
b) Position: flexed.
c) Station: at the level of the spines.
d) Engagement: two-fifths.
e) Presenting part: shoulder.

Maternal and perinatal mortality: the confidential enquiry

3   **Maternal mortality:**
a) Includes death caused by an ectopic pregnancy.
b) Is subjected to a confidential enquiry.
c) Must be reported to the Coroner.
d) Epilepsy is the commonest cause of indirect maternal death.
e) Is most often caused by sepsis.

4 Confidential Enquiry into Stillbirths and Deaths in Infancy (CESDI):
a) Includes only deaths after 24 weeks.
b) Late neonatal deaths occur after the first month of life.
c) The principal cause of death in the last CESDI was congenital abnormality.
d) Was set up to investigate suboptimal medical care.
e) Perinatal death: all stillbirths plus deaths in the first week of life.

Conception, implantation and embryology

5 During development of the ovarian follicles:
a) The primary oocyte is arrested at the interphase of the second meiotic division.
b) Granulosa cells in the corpus luteum are responsible for steroidogenesis.
c) Theca cells produce testosterone from cholesterol.
d) Meiosis is resumed prior to the luteinizing hormone (LH) surge.
e) The first polar body is extruded prior to ovulation.

6 After a successful conception the following statements are true:
a) The embryo remains in the fallopian tube for 6–8 days.
b) Myometrial cytokines modulate cytotrophoblastic proteolytic activity.
c) At 11 days the implantation site can be seen as a red spot on the endometrial mucosa.
d) Human chorionic gonadotrophin is produced by the corpus luteum.
e) The embryonic disc is formed after the third week postfertilization.

7 Considering embryo development:
a) During the third week, the bilaminar embryo generates the mesoderm.
b) At day 28, the cephalic neuropore closes.
c) Cardiac activity is evident from day 26.
d) The lower respiratory system appears as septation of the foregut.
e) The fetus is recognizably human at 12 weeks' gestation.

Physiological changes in pregnancy

8 In normal pregnancy:
a) Blood pressure falls in the second trimester.
b) Plasma volume decreases throughout gestation.
c) There is a reduction in erythrocyte production.
d) 50 per cent of women have a transient diastolic murmur.
e) There is an increase in the number of polymorphonuclear leucocytes.

9 Maternal effects on the physiology of the kidney include:
a) There is a 40 per cent increase in renal blood flow.
b) There is an increase in the glomerular filtration rate.
c) The urea and creatinine are higher than the non-pregnant state.
d) The upper limit of protein excretion in pregnancy is 0.6 g per day.
e) The kidneys increase in size.

Normal fetal development

10 During lung development:
a) Alveolar development occurs after 20 weeks.
b) The predominant phospholipid is phosphatidylcholine.
c) Fetal lung fluid production ceases in the second stage of labour.
d) Fetal breathing movement occurs for 30 per cent in the second trimester.
e) The production of lecithin is enhanced by cortisol and diabetes.

Antenatal care

11 With regard to routine antenatal care:
a) There is no evidence in low-risk pregnancies that reduction in antenatal visits increase maternal or fetal mortality.
b) The Naegele rule states that the expected date of delivery (EDD) is calculated by adding 7 days to the last menstrual period (LMP) and then taking away 4 months.
c) Syphilis testing forms part of the routine booking visit.
d) Routine urine testing reduces preterm labour.
e) Every patient should have a named consultant.

12 The routine dating scan:
a) Allows accurate dating of the pregnancy and a reduction in induction of labour for prolonged pregnancy.
b) Allows the detection of placenta praevia.
c) Allows early detection of twin pregnancies.
d) Allows detection of a failed pregnancy.
e) Allows detection of uterine abnormalities.

Antenatal imaging and fetal assessment

13 Regarding diagnostic ultrasound:
a) It employs the use of low-frequency, high-intensity sound waves.
b) Between 12 and 20 weeks, the crown–rump length and femur length are the most reproducible assessment of gestational age.
c) It can be used to determine chorionicity accurately in twin pregnancy at the 20-week scan.
d) It has shown that an increased nuchal translucency is associated with cardiac defects.
e) In 6 per cent of pregnancies, there will be a serious fetal structural abnormality.

14 Considering Doppler ultrasound:
a) Abnormal uterine Doppler flow indicates fetal hypoxaemia.
b) Abnormal umbilical artery flow indicates poor placental perfusion.
c) Fetal anaemia is associated with redistribution of blood flow.
d) Fetal hypoxaemia is associated with hyperdynamic circulation.
e) Abnormal ductus venosus blood flow occurs prior to arterial changes.

15 In relation to normal cardiotocograms at term:
a) The baseline at term is usually 120–160 beats per minute.
b) The baseline variability is considered abnormal when it is <10 beats per minute.
c) An acceleration is a baseline increase of 15 beats per minute for 15 seconds.
d) A reactive trace would have one acceleration in 20 minutes.
e) The tocograph trace indicates the strength of the contractions.

Prenatal diagnosis

16 The following statements are true for prenatal tests:
a) Serum biochemistry is superior to maternal age as a screening test for Down's syndrome.
b) Maternal serum alpha-fetoprotein is a diagnostic test for neural tube defects.
c) Amniocentesis has a higher pregnancy loss rate than chorionic villus sampling.
d) Tests using DNA technology can be performed on amniocentesis specimens.
e) Chorionic villus sampling can only be performed before 12 weeks' gestation.

17 Considering neural tube defects:
a) These occur as a result of poor preconception maternal diet.
b) The majority of these defects occur at the cranial end of the spine.
c) The prognosis for spina bifida depends on the level of the lesion.
d) With a previously affected sibling, the recurrence risk is 1 per cent.
e) A supplement of 4 mg folic acid significantly reduces the risk of recurrence.

Second trimester miscarriage

18 Second trimester miscarriage:
a) Is typically painless.
b) Occurs between 12 and 24 weeks' gestation.
c) Can be associated with rupture of the fetal membranes.
d) Is diagnosed after exclusion of infection, haemorrhage and multiple pregnancy.
e) Antibiotic prophylaxis is usually given.

Antenatal obstetric complications

19 Oligohydramnios is associated with the following fetal conditions:
a) Tracheo-oesophageal fistula.
b) Talipes.
c) Intrauterine growth restriction.
d) Anecephaly.
e) Premature rupture of the fetal membranes.

20 Polyhydramnios is associated with the following:
a) Maternal diabetes.
b) Neuromuscular fetal conditions.
c) Maternal non-steroidal anti-inflammatory drugs.
d) Postmaturity.
e) Chorioangioma of the placenta.

Twins and higher order multiple gestations

21 In twin delivery:
a) The first twin is at greater risk then the second.
b) Cephalic–cephalic presentation is the most common.
c) Labour usually occurs prior to term.
d) Labour is extended.
e) There is a risk of postpartum haemorrhage.

22 **Multiple pregnancies predispose to:**
a) Placenta praevia.
b) Diabetes mellitus.
c) Pre-eclampsia.
d) Malpresentation.
e) Intrauterine growth restriction (IUGR).

Disorders of placentation

23 **With regard to the placenta:**
a) It receives the highest blood flow of any fetal organ.
b) It has approximately 20 cotelydons.
c) The maternal and fetal blood are separated by one layer.
d) It is a major endocrine organ.
e) Each cotelydon contains a primary stem villus.

24 **Pre-eclampsia is more common in:**
a) Multigravid women.
b) Women with congenital cardiac disease.
c) Multiple pregnancy.
d) Women with diabetes insipidus.
e) Women with pre-existing renal disease.

25 **The treatment of pre-eclampsia includes:**
a) Hospital admission.
b) Labetolol.
c) Early delivery.
d) Frusemide.
e) Magnesium sulphate.

Preterm labour

26 **The following drugs have been shown to be effective in the treatment of preterm labour:**
a) Atosiban.
b) Pethidine.
c) Nifedipine.
d) Labetolol.
e) Ritodrine.

Medical diseases of pregnancy

27 **The risks of premature preterm rupture of the fetal membranes include:**
a) Premature labour.
b) Cord prolapse.
c) Pre-eclampsia.
d) Maternal septicaemia.
e) Antepartum haemorrhage.

28 **Women with congenital heart disease:**
a) Should have a detailed fetal cardiology scan.
b) Should avoid becoming anaemic.
c) Should have prophylactic antibiotics for operative deliveries.
d) Commonly develop dysrhythmias.
e) Should have a shortened second stage of labour.

29 **Hyperthyroidism in pregnancy:**
a) Should be treated surgically rather than with carbimazole.
b) Can be diagnosed by total T4 measurements.
c) 50 per cent are secondary to Graves' disease.
d) The main complications for the fetus include growth restriction and fetal bradycardia.
e) Therapy should maintain free T4 and T3 levels in the low normal range.

30 **Patients diagnosed as having mitral stenosis:**
a) Usually have been diagnosed prior to pregnancy.
b) Account for 50 per cent of rheumatic heart problems.
c) Should have an elective Caesarean section at 38–39 weeks.
d) Should be considered for mitral valvotomy during pregnancy.
e) Should not be given ergometrine routinely for the third stage.

31 **The infant of a diabetic mother is at increased risk of:**
a) Polycythemia.
b) Hypermagnesaemia.
c) Traumatic delivery.
d) Neonatal jaundice.
e) Hypoglycaemia.

32 **Addison's disease:**
a) Is usually an autoimmune process.
b) Is not an indication for Caesarean section.
c) Has no effect on the fetus.
d) Carries a good prognosis in pregnancy.
e) Diagnosis in pregnancy is difficult owing to high oestrogen levels.

33 **Considering cystic fibrosis in pregnancy:**
a) The partner does not need genetic testing.
b) This is an autosomal recessive disorder.
c) The woman should have an oral glucose tolerance test.
d) Caesarean section is mandatory owing to poor lung function.
e) Fetal growth should be monitored with serial ultrasound scanning.

34 **With reference to iron deficiency anaemia in pregnancy:**
a) Iron demand in pregnancy increases to 4 mg per day.
b) High levels of serum ferritin confirm the diagnosis.
c) It is more common in multiple pregnancy.
d) It is usually be treated with oral iron.
e) Blood transfusion should be avoided.

35 Regarding thalassaemias:
a) They represent the commonest genetic disorder.
b) They result from an amino-acid substitution.
c) Alpha-thalassaemia major is incompatible with intrauterine life.
d) It is important to screen the partner.
e) Beta-thalassaemia minor is not a problem antenatally.

36 Intrahepatic cholestasis in pregnancy is associated with:
a) Elevation of total bile salts in the blood.
b) A positive direct Coombs' test in the neonate.
c) Neonatal jaundice.
d) Intrapartum fetal distress.
e) Marked geographical variations.

37 In relation to women who embark on pregnancy with a diagnosis of epilepsy:
a) Carbamazepine is associated with neural tube defects.
b) Postpartum antiepileptic drugs may need to be reduced.
c) Vitamin K should be commenced from 30 weeks' gestation.
d) Women on multiple therapy should be converted to monotherapy.
e) Intravenous magnesium sulphate is the best treatment of a status epilepticus during labour.

Perinatal infections

38 With regard to congenital infection with cytomegalovirus:
a) It is characterized by intracerebral calcification.
b) It is a recognized cause of microcephaly.
c) It can be detected by culture of the infant's urine.
d) It is a cause of developmental delay.
e) 90 per cent of infections are asymptomatic.

39 Congenital malformation can be attributed to maternal infection with:
a) Poliomyelitis.
b) Toxoplasmosis.
c) Measles.
d) Parvovirus.
e) Syphilis.

40 Considering human immunodeficiency virus:
a) It is a retrovirus.
b) The antibody test may take 1 month to become positive after exposure.
c) The vertical transmission rate is approximately 15 per cent.
d) Stopping breast feeding is an effective way of preventing vertical transmission.
e) With intervention, the vertical transmission rate can be reduced to 3 per cent.

Labour

41 With regard to anatomy of the maternal pelvis:
a) The pudendal nerve passes in front of the ischial spine.
b) The anterior–posterior diameter of the pelvic inlet is 11 cm.
c) The anterior–posterior diameter of the pelvic outlet is 11 cm.
d) The levator ani muscles form the pelvic floor.
e) The angle of the inlet to the horizontal can be up to 90°.

42 Considering the fetal skull:
a) The anterior fontenelle is diamond shaped.
b) The sutures of the vault are ossified.
c) The vertex presentation longitudinal diameter is the subocciptal–frontal diameter.
d) The occipito-mental diameter is normally too large to pass through the maternal pelvis.
e) Moulding of the fetal skull is a normal physiological process.

43 Progress in labour is measured by:
a) The frequency of uterine contractions.
b) The force of uterine contractions.
c) Descent of the presenting part.
d) Dilation of the cervix.
e) The length of time since rupture of the membranes.

44 In relation to the mechanism of labour:
a) Engagement is said to have occurred when the widest part of the presenting part has passed through the false pelvis.
b) Restitution occurs after external rotation.
c) Extension occurs after internal rotation.
d) Extension occurs at 'crowning'.
e) Descent of the fetal head is needed before flexion, internal rotation and extension can occur.

45 Regarding face presentation:
a) This occurs in 1:250 labours.
b) The presenting diameter is the submento-bregmatic, which is 9.5 cm.
c) It is commonly due to fetal thyroid tumours.
d) The face can deliver vaginally with the chin meno-anterior.
e) Oxytocin should be used to augment slow progress.

46 Considering the Bishop's score:
a) It includes station of the presenting part.
b) It includes the length of the cervical canal.
c) It includes the gestation of the fetus.
d) It includes parity of the mother.
e) A score of 4 indicates the cervix is unfavourable.

47 Concerning brow presentation:
a) This may be treated in labour by craniotomy.
b) It is the least common malposition.
c) The presenting diameter is mento-vertical.
d) It may be treated in labour by Caesarean section.
e) This is incompatible with vaginal delivery.

48 The following are contraindications to epidural anaesthesia:
a) Previous treatment with coagulants.
b) Multiple pregnancy.
c) Lack of trained staff.
d) Hypertension in pregnancy.
e) Patients receiving narcotics.

49 Vaginal bleeding in the first stage of labour may be due to:
a) Placental abruption.
b) Cervical fibroids.
c) Ruptured uterus.
d) Vaginal trauma.
e) Vasa praevia.

Operative interventions in obstetrics

50 The advantages of the midline episiotomy are:
a) Less blood loss.
b) Reduced incidence of dyspareunia.
c) Less anal sphincter damage.
d) Less pain in the postpartum period.
e) It is easier to repair.

51 Kjelland's forceps:
a) Have a pelvic curvature.
b) Have a cephalic curvature.
c) Have a sliding lock.
d) Are used to rotate an occipital-posterior position.
e) Should not be used under pudendal block anaesthesia alone.

52 Indications and prerequisites for delivery with the ventouse include:
a) Delay in the second stage.
b) The cervix is fully dilated.
c) Gestation less than 34 weeks.
d) Fetal distress in the second stage.
e) Fetal membranes are ruptured.

53 During an assisted breech delivery:
a) An episiotomy can be cut once the anus is seen at the fourchette.
b) Pinard's manoeuvre can be used to deliver legs in the extended position.
c) Mauriceau–Smellie–Veit's manoeuvre is used to deliver extended arms.
d) Forceps should not be applied to the fetal head.
e) Epidural analgesia is mandatory.

54 The following complications are more likely after Caesarean section than after vaginal delivery:
a) Pulmonary embolism.
b) Secondary postpartum haemorrhage.
c) Postnatal depression.
d) Amniotic fluid embolism.
e) Infection.

Obstetric emergencies

55 With regard to shoulder dystocia:
a) It occurs in approximately 1 per cent of labours.
b) It is more common in assisted vaginal delivery.
c) McRobert's manoeuvre will be effective in 90 per cent of cases.
d) Fundal pressure should be avoided.
e) Avoid lateral flexion of the head on the neck.

The puerperium

56 Human milk has the following advantages over formula milk:
a) Human milk contains more protein.
b) Human milk contains more lactose.
c) Human milk is associated with a reduction in atopic illness.
d) Human milk is a good source of iron.
e) Human milk is a good source of vitamin K.

Psychiatric disorders in pregnancy and the puerperium

57 Postnatal blues:
a) Usually start between days 3 and 5.
b) May be prolonged by anaemia.
c) Are more common in women who have normal deliveries.
d) Are prevented by night sedation.
e) Occur in women who are discharged early for hospital.

Neonatology

58 Neonatal jaundice is a recognized feature of:
a) Sickle cell disease.
b) Glucose-6-phosphate dehydrogenase.
c) Rhesus incompatibility.
d) Beta-thalassaemia.
e) Meningitis.

59 The following are thought to protect against hyaline membrane disease in the neonate:
a) Intrauterine growth restriction.
b) Severe pre-eclampsia.
c) Heroin addiction.
d) Prolonged rupture of the fetal membranes.
e) Diabetes mellitus.

MCQ answers

1 **True: c, d.** Pregnancy is dated from the last menstrual period. Gravidity is the total number of pregnancies regardless of how they ended. Domestic violence is an increasing problem and it is recommended that all women are seen on their own to discuss this potential problem. A family history of pre-eclampsia increases the risk pre-eclampsia in this pregnancy.
See Chapter 1, *Obstetrics by Ten Teachers*, 18th edition.

2 **True: c, d, e.** Cephalic describes presentation and not lie. The shoulder presents with a transverse lie.
See Chapter 1, *Obstetrics by Ten Teachers*, 18th edition.

3 **True: a, b.** Maternal death is defined as the death of a woman while pregnant or within 42 days of termination of pregnancy, from any cause related to or aggravated by the pregnancy or its management, but not from accidental or incidental causes. The commonest indirect cause of maternal death is cardiac disease, with suicide as the next most common. The commonest cause of maternal death on the last confidential enquiry was thromboembolic disease.
See Chapter 3, *Obstetrics by Ten Teachers*, 18th edition.

4 **True: d, e.** CESDI applies to deaths after 20 weeks' gestation. The definition of late neonatal is death from 7 to 27 completed days after delivery. The principal cause of fetal death is prematurity and not congenital abnormality. The report classifies cases according to the type of care that they received.
See Chapter 3, *Obstetrics by Ten Teachers*, 18th edition.

5 **True: b, c, e.** The primary oocyte is arrested at the metaphase of the second meiotic division and not the interphase of the cycle. Meiosis is not resumed until after the LH surge. The first polar body is extruded prior to ovulation and the second polar body is extruded after ovulation.
See Chapter 4, *Obstetrics by Ten Teachers*, 18th edition.

6 **True: c.** The embryo after fertilization remains in the fallopian tube for 3–4 days. It is endometrial cytokines not myometrial cytokines that modulate cytotrophoblastic proteolytic activity to control the depth of invasion. Human chorionic gonadotrophin is produced by the trophoblast; therefore, it is a specific indicator of pregnancy. It can also be utilized in the diagnosis of ectopic pregnancy. The embryonic period starts with the generation of the embryonic disc during the second week postfertilization.
See Chapter 4, *Obstetrics by Ten Teachers*, 18th edition.

7 **True: a, d, e.** The cephalic neuropore closes during the 26th day and the caudal neuropore on the 28th day after fertilization. Cardiac activity is evident from day 22.
See Chapter 4, *Obstetrics by Ten Teachers*, 18th edition.

8 **True: a, e.** The plasma volume increases in pregnancy until around 32 weeks after which time it plateaus. The increase in the plasma volume is one of the fundamental physiological changes of normal pregnancy. This change is essential to other physiological changes that occur during pregnancy, which include increased cardiac output and an increase in renal blood flow. Erythrocyte production is increased in pregnancy; however, there is marked dilution of red cells in the blood owing to the increased plasma volume. The maternal heart sounds change during pregnancy: there is an increased loudness in both s1 and s2, >95 per cent of women develop a systolic murmur that disappears after delivery, and 20 per cent have a transient diastolic murmur.
See Chapter 5, *Obstetrics by Ten Teachers*, 18th edition.

9 **True: b, e.** During pregnancy, there is a dramatic (60–75 per cent) increase in the renal blood flow. The consequence of this is an increase in the glomerular filtration rate (GFR) of the kidney. The increase in the GFR is responsible for an increase in the clearance of urea and creatinine. Thus plasma concentrations of urea and creatinine are reduced during pregnancy. Kidneys increase in length by approximately 1 cm during pregnancy.
See Chapter 5, *Obstetrics by Ten Teachers*, 18th edition.

10 **True: b.** The fetal alveoli start to develop after 20 weeks' gestation. The predominant phospholipid is phosphatidylcholine (lecithin). The production of lecithin is enhanced by cortisol, growth restriction and prolonged rupture of membranes. However, diabetes mellitus delays the production of respiratory lecithin. The fetal lung is filled with fluid from an early gestation. Its production ceases in the early stages of labour under the influence of adrenaline.
See Chapter 6, *Obstetrics by Ten Teachers*, 18th edition.

11 **True: a, c.** The Naegele rule states that the EDD is calculated by adding 7 days to the LMP and then taking away 3 months. However, this rule assumes a 28-day cycle and ovulation on day 14, and finally an accurate recollection of the LMP. Although only a small number of women are diagnosed with syphilis during pregnancy, the vertical transmission to the fetus has serious consequences. This transmission to the fetus can easily be prevented by treatment of the mother with antibiotics. There are several classifications of antenatal care; if the women have community care, then the lead clinician would be the community midwife.
See Chapter 7, *Obstetrics by Ten Teachers*, 18th edition.

12 **True: a, c, d, e.** The routine dating scan is unable to detect placenta praevia. Placenta praevia can be detected by ultrasound but not until the third trimester.
See Chapter 7, *Obstetrics by Ten Teachers*, 18th edition.

13 **True: d.** The technique of ultrasound utilizes high-frequency, low-intensity sound waves to generate an image. Fetal age can be assessed accurately prior to 12 weeks by measuring the crown–rump length and from 12 to 20 weeks gestation can be determined from biparental diameter. The chorionicity of twin pregnancy is best determined in the first trimester; this should ideally occur at approximately 12 weeks. Nuchal translucency has been shown to be a screening test for Down's syndrome, other chromosomal abnormalities and cardiac defects. Serious fetal structural abnormalities are diagnosed in 3 per cent of all pregnancies.
See Chapter 8, *Obstetrics by Ten Teachers*, 18th edition.

14 **True: b.** Abnormal uterine artery Doppler indices are used as indicators for an increased risk of pre-eclampsia and intrauterine fetal growth restriction. Fetal anaemia is associated with a hyperdynamic circulation, whereas fetal hypoxaemia is associated with blood redistribution. Abnormal flow in the ductus venosus is a pre-terminal observation and does not precede arterial changes.
See Chapter 8, *Obstetrics by Ten Teachers*, 18th edition.

15 **True: b, c.** The normal fetal heart rate at term is 110–150 beats per minute, whilst prior to term 160 beats per minute is taken as the upper limit of normal. Normal baseline variability reflects a normal fetal autonomic nervous system. Baseline variability is considered abnormal when less than 10 beats per minute. The presence of two or more accelerations on 20–30-minute cardiotocogram defines a reactive trace.
See Chapter 8, *Obstetrics by Ten Teachers*, 18th edition.

16 **True: a, d.** Serum biochemistry has a sensitivity of 60–70 per cent, compared to 30–40 per cent for maternal age alone. The measurement of serum alpha-fetoprotein is a screening test for neural tube defects and not a diagnostic test. Chorionic villus biopsy is usually performed between 11 weeks' and 20 weeks' gestation.
See Chapter 9, *Obstetrics by Ten Teachers*, 18th edition.

17 **True: b, c, e.** Neural tube defects (NTDs) are amongst the common major abnormalities. The aetiology is multifactorial with well-defined environmental, genetic, pharmacological and geographical factors implicated. Around 70–80 per cent of neural tube defects are anencephaly or encephaloceles. When a parent or previous sibling has had an NTD, the risk of recurrence is 5–10 per cent. Preconception folate supplementation of the

maternal diet reduces the risk of developing these defects by about half. The dosage of folic acid is 400 μ g for primary prevention and 4 mg for women wishing to prevent a recurrence of an NTD.
See Chapter 9, *Obstetrics by Ten Teachers*, 18th edition.

18 **True: b, c.** Second trimester miscarriage normally presents with backache, contractions and vaginal bleeding. Rupture of the fetal membranes can also be a feature. Antibiotics are only given if there is strong evidence there is infection.
See Chapter 10, *Obstetrics by Ten Teachers*, 18th edition.

19 **True: b, c, e.** Tracheo-oesophageal fistula and anecephaly are both associated with polyhydramnios due to lack of fetal swallowing.
See Chapter 11, *Obstetrics by Ten Teachers*, 18th edition.

20 **True: a, b, e.** Postmaturity is associated with oligohydramnios.
See Chapter 11 *Obstetrics by Ten Teachers*, 18th edition.

21 **True: b, c, e.** It has been shown that the fetal mortality and morbidity are greatest in the second twin. The labour is of normal length.
See Chapter 12, *Obstetrics by Ten Teachers*, 18th edition.

22 **True: a, c, d, e.** The greater placental area makes placenta praevia more likely. Acute pyelonephritis, IUGR, hypertension, polyhydramnios, malpresentation and prematurity are more common in multiple pregnancies.
See Chapter 12, *Obstetrics by Ten Teachers*, 18th edition.

23 **True: a, b, c, e.** It receives the highest flow of any fetal organ and towards the end of pregnancy, competes with the fetus for maternal substrate, consuming the major fraction of glucose and oxygen taken up by the gravid uterus. The functional unit of the placenta is the cotyledon, and the mature human placenta has about 20 cotyledons. The septa, which divide the placenta into its cotyledons, appear at the end of the third month of development. Three microscopic tissue layers separate the maternal and fetal blood: the trophoblast tissue, connective tissue and the endothelium.
See Chapter 13, *Obstetrics by Ten Teachers*, 18th edition.

24 **True: c, e.** Pre-eclampsia is more common in primagravid women, women with diabetes mellitus (not diabetes insipidus) and in women with pre-existing renal disease.
See Chapter 13, *Obstetrics by Ten Teachers*, 18th edition.

25 **True: b, c, d, e.** Hospital admission is not a treatment for the condition; however, it allows the severity of the condition to be quantified via continuous assessment of the blood pressure and serial haematological and biochemical parameters. Delivery will cure the condition. In pre-eclampsia, the plasma volume is reduced; therefore, frusemide will not help and may make matters worse.
See Chapter 13, *Obstetrics by Ten Teachers*, 18th edition.

26 **True: a, c, e.** Ritodrine is a sympathomimetic and causes uterine relaxation. Nifedipine can be used to arrest preterm delivery as it acts to inhibit intracellular calcium. Atosiban is a specific oxytocin receptor antagonist and, therefore, reduces uterine contractions. Labetolol is an alpha- and beta-receptor agonist used in the reduction of blood pressure. Pethidine sedates the mother and the fetus but does not affect the contractions.
See Chapter 14, *Obstetrics by Ten Teachers*, 18th edition.

27 **True: a, b, d.** The risks are premature labour, malpresentation, cord prolapse and ascending infections. Any women delivering after preterm rupture of the fetal membranes is at risk of postpartum haemorrhage and endometritis.
See Chapter 14, *Obstetrics by Ten Teachers*, 18th edition.

28 **True: a, b, c, e.** The incidence of congenital heart disease in the general population is 8 per 1000 live births. However, if the parent is affected, the incidence raises to 5 per 100 live births; therefore, all pregnant women

with congenital heart disease should have a detailed fetal cardiology scan. The haemodynamic changes of pregnancy increase the strain on the heart. Anaemia exacerbates this situation. Dysrhythmias occur in less than 3 per cent of women. However, they require urgent treatment. Prophylactic antibiotics should be given to any women with congenital heart defects.
See Chapter 15, *Obstetrics by Ten Teachers*, 18th edition.

29 **None are true.** The treatment of hyperthyroidism in pregnancy is drug treatment. Radioactive iodine is completely contraindicated owing to its effect on the fetal thyroid gland. Surgical treatment may be rarely indicated where there is no response to medical therapy. During pregnancy, there is an increase in the levels of total T4 and T3; however, there is no increase in the levels of the free hormones. Therefore, the diagnosis requires increased levels of free T4 and T3, and reduced levels of thyroid-stimulating hormone. Approximately 90 per cent are due to Graves' disease. The main complications for the fetus include fetal growth restriction, stillbirth, fetal tachycardia and premature delivery.
See Chapter 15, *Obstetrics by Ten Teachers*, 18th edition.

30 **True: a, e.** Most cases of heart disease are diagnosed prior to pregnancy. Mitral stenosis is the commonest acquired cardiac lesion, accounting for 90 per cent of rheumatic problems. Mitral valvotomy can be performed during pregnancy, if necessary.
See Chapter 15, *Obstetrics by Ten Teachers*, 18th edition.

31 **True: a, c ,d , e.** The infant of a diabetic mother is at increased risk of various metabolic and traumatic insults. The fetus is at increased risk of hypoglycaemia, hypocalcaemia, hypomagnesaemia.
See Chapter 15, *Obstetrics by Ten Teachers*, 18th edition.

32 **True: a, b, c, d.** The diagnosis can be difficult in pregnancy because of cortisol levels; instead of being characteristically reduced, they may be in the low normal range.
See Chapter 15, *Obstetrics by Ten Teachers*, 18th edition.

33 **True: b, c, e.** It is important to test the partner for carrier status so that an accurate assessment of fetal risk can be made. The couple should be offered genetic counselling regarding the risk of the fetus having cystic fibrosis or being a carrier. Pancreatic function is affected in women with cystic fibrosis and 8 per cent will develop gestational diabetes in pregnancy. Ideally, vaginal delivery should be the aim; however, the second stage may be shortened in the event of maternal exhaustion. The fetal risks include fetal growth restriction.
See Chapter 15, *Obstetrics by Ten Teachers*, 18th edition.

34 **True: a, c, d.** Iron demand in pregnancy increases from 2 to 4 mg daily. The diagnosis of iron deficiency is suspected if the mean corpuscular volume (MCV) is below 85 fL. Low levels of serum iron and ferritin help to confirm the diagnosis. Nutritional status affects the iron stores, and repeated pregnancy and poor social factors may lead to anaemia as will the increased iron requirements of multiple pregnancy. Blood transfusion should be avoided, if possible, because of the small risk of antibody production and transfusion reaction.
See Chapter 15, *Obstetrics by Ten Teachers*, 18th edition.

35 **True: a, c, d, e.** The genetic defect in thalassaemia causes a reduced production of normal haemoglobin, whereas sickle cell disease is caused by an amino-acid substitution that results in it precipitating when in its reduced state. Alpha-thalassaemia major is incompatible with intrauterine life, with the fetus developing marked hydrops.
See Chapter 15, *Obstetrics by Ten Teachers*, 18th edition.

36 **True: a, d, e.** In intrahepatic cholestasis (IHC), the serum shows an increase in conjugated bilirubin and alkaline phosphatase. There is large geographical variation in the incidence of IHC with one of the highest incidences occurring in Chile. The fetal risks for obstetric cholestasis include preterm labour, meconium staining and, rarely, intrauterine fetal death.
See Chapter 15, *Obstetrics by Ten Teachers*, 18th edition.

37 **True : a, b, d.** Carbamazepine is classically associated with neural tube defects. However, sodium valproate is associated with NTDs, genitourinary and cardiac defects, and phenytoin is associated with cardiac and genitourinary defects. Vitamin K supplementation should be recommended from 36 weeks' gestation. This is because vitamin K-dependent clotting factors within the newborn may be reduced and lead to haemorrhagic disease. Although magnesium sulphate is the treatment of choice for an undiagnosed seizure during labour, intravenous benzodiazipines (i.e. lorazepam, carbamazepine) are the recognized treatment for status epilepticus during labour.
See Chapter 15, *Obstetrics by Ten Teachers*, 18th edition.

38 **All are true.** Congenital cytomegalovirus (CMV) is associated with various fetal manifestations. These include hepatosplenomegaly, microcephaly, intrauterine growth retardation, hyperbilirubinaemia, intracerebral calcification and mental retardation. Only 5–10 per cent of infants will be symptomatic at birth. Congenital CMV is a cause of fetal hydrops and, as such, polyhydramnios.
See Chapter 16, *Obstetrics by Ten Teachers*, 18th edition.

39 **True: b, e.** Toxoplasmosis during the first trimester of pregnancy is mostly likely to cause fetal damage, but only 10–25 per cent are transmitted to the fetus. In the third trimester, 75–90 per cent of infections are transmitted, but the risk of fetal damage in almost zero at term. Up to 70 per cent of fetuses become infected if the mother has primary or secondary syphilis during pregnancy; however, the spectrum of congenital disease varies greatly.
See Chapter 16, *Obstetrics by Ten Teachers*, 18th edition.

40 **All are true.** Human immunodeficiency virus (HIV) is a retrovirus, with the genetic code in a single strand of RNA. Vertical transmission occurs in 25–40 per cent of pregnancies where there is no intervention to reduce the risk. Three interventions have been shown to reduce the vertical transmission of HIV. These are: (1) avoiding breastfeeding; (2) elective Caesarean section; and (3) antiviral medication during the latter half of pregnancy. If all three interventions are undertaken, then the risk of transmission is probably less than 3 per cent.
See Chapter 16, *Obstetrics by Ten Teachers*, 18th edition.

41 **True: b, d, e.** The pudendal nerve passes behind and below the ischial spine. The pelvic inlet is defined as the area bounded in front by the symphysis pubis, on each side by the upper margin of the pubic bone, the ileopectineal line and the ala of the sacrum, and posteriorly by the promontory of the sacrum. The normal anterior–posterior (AP) diameter of the pelvic inlet is 11 cm and the transverse diameter is 13.5 cm. The AP diameter of the pelvic outlet is 13.5 cm, with a transverse diameter of 11 cm. The normal angle of the inlet is 60° to the horizontal, however, in Afro-Caribbean women, this angle may be as much as 90°.
See Chapter 17, *Obstetrics by Ten Teachers*, 18th edition.

42 **True: a, d, e.** The anterior fontanelle is diamond shaped and is formed at the junction of the sagittal, frontal and coronal sutures. The sutures of the vault are soft unossified membranes, whereas the sutures of the face and the skull base are firmly united. The longitudinal diameter of the vertex presentation is the suboccipital–bregmatic diameter. The occipito-mental diameter is 13 cm and describes the brow presentation. This is usually too large to pass through the maternal pelvis.
See Chapter 17, *Obstetrics by Ten Teachers*, 18th edition.

43 **True: c, d.** Progress is measured by the dilatation of the cervix and the descent of the presenting part. It may be satisfactory in the absence of strong frequent contractions or may appear unsatisfactory even when the contractions are strong.
See Chapter 17, *Obstetrics by Ten Teachers*, 18th edition.

44 **True: c, d, e.** Engagement is said to have occurred when the widest part of the presenting part has passed through the pelvic inlet. Restitution occurs directly after delivery of the fetal head, this allows the fetal head to align itself with the shoulders in the oblique position. In order to deliver, the shoulders then have to rotate

from the oblique into the AP plane. During this rotation, the fetal occiput rotates to the transverse and this is termed external rotation.
See Chapter 17, *Obstetrics by Ten Teachers,* 18th edition.

45 **True: b, d.** Face presentation occurs in about 1 in 500 labours. Rarely, extension of the neck can due to a fetal anomaly, such as a thyroid tumour. If progress in labour is excellent, and the chin remains mento-anterior, vaginal delivery is possible by flexion. Oxytocin should not be used and, if there are any concerns about fetal condition, Caesarean section should be carried out.
See Chapter 17, *Obstetrics by Ten Teachers,* 18th edition.

46 **True: a, b, e.** Bishop's score relates to the favourability of the cervix for induction of labour. It scores the station of the presenting part, the cervical consistency, position, dilation and effacement. High scores are associated with an easier shorter induction that is less likely to fail. Low scores are associated with longer inductions of labour, which are more likely to fail and result in Caesarean section.
See Chapter 17, *Obstetrics by Ten Teachers,* 18th edition.

47 **True: c, d.** Brow presentation is the least common *malpresentation* (1 in 1500) not malposition. Malposition refers to the abnormal position of the occiput in a vertex presentation. The presenting diameter is mento-vertical (measuring 13.5 cm). This is incompatible with a vaginal delivery.
See Chapter 17, *Obstetrics by Ten Teachers,* 18th edition.

48 **True: c.** Coagulation disorders are a contraindication to epidural anaesthesia; however, previous use of coagulants is not an indication. Lack of trained staff is a contraindication to the use of epidural analgesia, as it may place patients at risk.
See Chapter 17, *Obstetrics by Ten Teachers,* 18th edition.

49 **True: a, c, e.** Any cause of antepartum haemorrhage may cause bleeding in the first stage of labour, including a late presenting placenta praevia or an intrapartum abruption. To these must be added conditions usually occurring in the first stage of labour. Vaginal trauma usually occurs in the second stage of labour with delivery of the fetal head.
See Chapter 17, *Obstetrics by Ten Teachers,* 18th edition.

50 **True: a, b, d, e.** The major disadvantage that it carries is a more than six-fold risk of it extending to involve the anal sphincter.
See Chapter 18, *Obstetrics by Ten Teachers,* 18th edition.

51 **True: b, c, e.** Kjelland's forceps have a cephalic curvature but no pelvic curvature. The sliding lock is used to correct asynclitsim. They should not be applied to a high head: one that is more than one-fifth palpable abdominally. The minimum analgesia requirement for delivery by Kjelland's forceps is an effective epidural or a spinal block. Kjelland's forceps should only be used by an experienced operator.
See Chapter 18, *Obstetrics by Ten Teachers,* 18th edition.

52 **True: a, b, d, e.** The maternal indication for assisted vaginal delivery are maternal exhaustion, maternal illness, where the Valsalva manoeuvre is contraindicated, and failure to descend owing to soft tissue resistance. Fetal indications include any condition that makes it unsafe for the fetus to remain in the uterus during second stage and a non-reassuring heart rate tracing. The prerequisites for instrumental delivery are adequate analgesia, empty bladder, cervix fully dilated, defined position and station, cephalic presentation and adequate uterus contraction.
See Chapter 18, *Obstetrics by Ten Teachers,* 18th edition.

53 **True: a, b,** An episiotomy should not be performed too early as heavy bleeding may occur but, once the fetal trunk is delivered, it is difficult to perform. Lovesett's manoeuvre is used to bring down extended arms. Mauriceau–Smellie–Veit's manoeuvre is used to deliver the aftercoming head of the breech in a controlled

manner; if this manoeuvre proves difficult, then obstetric forceps need to be applied to aid delivery of the fetal head.
See Chapter 18, *Obstetrics by Ten Teachers,* 18th edition.

54 **True: a, c, e.** Overall, the risks of both early and long-term complications are increased in women delivered by Caesarean section. The main problems are thromboembolism, infection and haemorrhage. Amniotic fluid embolism usually occurs during or immediately after labour and is no more common after Caesarean section. Secondary postpartum haemorrhage is usually due to retained products and is less common after section. Between 10 and 15 per cent of women will suffer with some form of depression in the first year after delivery of their baby and it is more common in women who have undergone a Caesarean section.
See Chapter 18, *Obstetrics by Ten Teachers,* 18th edition.

55 **All are true.** Difficulty with delivery of the fetal shoulder is termed shoulder dystocia. The incidence varies from between 0.2 to 1.2 per cent depending on the definition used. Risk factors for shoulder dystocia include large baby, small mother, maternal obesity, postmaturity and assisted vaginal delivery. Shoulder dystocia should be managed in a sequence of manoeuvres designed to facilitate delivery without fetal damage. The first of these manoeuvres is McRobert's manoeuvre (maximal flex and abduction of the patient's hips onto her abdomen) and this will effect safe delivery in approximately 90 per cent of cases. Fundal pressure should be avoided, as it may lead to rupture of the uterus. Inappropriate traction on the fetal head causing lateral flexion should be avoided, as this can result in nerve damage and Erd's palsy.
See Chapter 19, *Obstetrics by Ten Teachers,* 18th edition.

56 **True: b, c.** Human milk has a low iron concentration; however, the iron is absorbed more efficiently from human than from formula milks.
See Chapter 20, *Obstetrics by Ten Teachers,* 18th edition.

57 **True: a, b, d.**

58 **True: b, c, e.** Two-thirds of babies develop jaundice in the first week of life. Any visible jaundice in the first 24 hours must be urgently investigated and assumed to be haemolysis until proven otherwise. Sickle cell and beta-thalassaemia are not associated with neonatal jaundice.
See Chapter 22, *Obstetrics by Ten Teachers,* 18th edition.

59 **True: a, b, c, d.** All these conditions stress the fetus and promote surfactant production. Surfactant production is inhibited in diabetes.

Chapter 3

Short answer questions

Modern maternity care

1 Discuss how maternity care has changed since its inception.

The modern National Health Service (NHS) was established by an Act of Parliament in 1946. This bill instigated free maternity care for all women. (1 mark)

Antenatal care was perceived as beneficial, acceptable and available for all. This was reinforced by the finding that the perinatal mortality rate seemed to be inversely proportional to the number of antenatal visits. (2 marks)

The cooperation card was launched on the NHS maternity services the 1950s. This allowed a continuous record to be held by the mother and improved the communication between all health care professionals involved in the delivery of maternity care. (2 marks)

The advent of obstetric ultrasound brought with it a dramatic revolution in the antenatal care and screening for fetal anomalies. This has allowed early pregnancy viability and accurate dating of pregnancies. Improved technologies with ultrasound have given rise to fetal anomaly screening. (3 marks)

During the early 1950s, there was a move toward hospital confinement from home confinement. Home deliveries are now an infrequent event with a countrywide average of about 2 per cent. (2 marks)

Screening has formed part of antenatal care since its inception. There are discrepancies in the screening tests offered for various diseases including Down's syndrome. The National Screening Committee has been set up to improve screening standards. (2 marks)

See Chapter 2, *Obstetrics by Ten Teachers*, 18th edition.

Maternal and perinatal mortality: the confidential enquiry

2 Write short notes on maternal mortality, perinatal mortality and Confidential Enquiry into Stillbirths and Deaths in Infancy (CESDI).

Maternal mortality

This can be defined as the death of a woman while pregnant, or within 42 days of the termination of pregnancy, from any cause related to, or aggravated by, the pregnancy or its management, but not from accidental or incidental causes. In the UK, this is the number of deaths from obstetric causes per 100 000 maternities.　　(2 marks)

This can be further subdivided into direct and indirect deaths. Direct deaths are those resulting from an obstetric complication, the most common being thromboembolism and hypertensive disorders.　　(2 marks)

Indirect deaths are those resulting from a previous existing disease or disease that developed during pregnancy and which is not due to a direct obstetric cause. The most common causes of indirect death are cardiac disease and psychiatric disorders.　　(2 marks)

Perinatal mortality

This is defined as the number of stillbirths and early neonatal deaths per 1000 live births and stillbirths.　　(2 marks)

The most common cause of death is antenatal fetal death, of this a quarter is unexplained, a quarter is associated with intrauterine growth retardation, and the remainder are associated with placental abruption and diabetes.　　(1 mark)

The next most common cause of death is immaturity. Although only 8 per cent of babies are born prematurely, this group comprises 50 per cent of all neonatal deaths. The immediate causes of death amongst this group include respiratory distress syndrome and neurological causes.　　(2 marks)

CESDI

This enquiry was set up in the early 1990s to improve the understanding of how the risk of death from 20 weeks of pregnancy to 1 year after birth might be reduced.　　(2 marks)

All deaths are notified to the regional coordinator so the full clinical picture can be obtained. A specialist panel will review only a subset of the cases. Each panel consists of experts from several disciplines, including an obstetrician, a paediatrician, a perinatal pathologist, a general practitioner and an independent chair. The panel grade the cases from 0 to 3. Grade 0 equates to no substandard care and 3 to suboptimal care, and a change in management would be expected to alter the outcome.　　(3 marks)

See Chapter 3, *Obstetrics by Ten Teachers*, 18th edition.

Physiological changes in pregnancy

3 Outline the physiological changes that occur in response to pregnancy in the cardiovascular system, the cervix and the respiratory system.

Cardiovascular system

Early pregnancy is characterized by a decrease in the peripheral vascular resistance. A significant increase in the heart rate is observed as early as 5 weeks, and this contributes to an increase in cardiac output. This increase in heart rate continues into the third trimester. The stroke volume increases in the late first trimester and further increases the cardiac output.　　(4 marks)

Cervix

Under the influence of the pregnancy hormones oestradiol and progesterone, the cervix becomes swollen and softer during pregnancy. Oestradiol stimulates the growth of the columnar epithelium of the cervical canal and this becomes visualized as an ectopy. Increased vascularity of the cervix causes it to become a blueish colour. Prostaglandins induce remodelling of the cervical collagen towards term, which allows softening.   (4 marks)

Respiratory system

Dramatic changes occur in the respiratory system with the onset of pregnancy. The increased cardiac output causes a substantial increase in the pulmonary blood flow. There is an increase in the tidal volume. These two effects combine to give more efficient oxygen exchange. This increase oxygen exchange causes a decrease in pCO_2 and a slight increase in pO_2. Thus oxygen availability to the tissues increases. The mechanical changes that occur in the lung include increases in the tidal volume, and decreases in the vital capacity and functional residual capacity.   (4 marks)

See Chapter 5, *Obstetrics by Ten Teachers*, 18th edition.

Normal fetal development

4 Write short notes on the fetal cardiovascular system and fetal blood.

Fetal cardiovascular system

The fetal circulation is significantly different from that of the adult. The lungs do not participate in oxygen exchange; therefore, their blood supply is significantly reduced. This reduction is achieved via the ductus arteriosus, which shunts blood away from the pulmonary artery and into the aorta.   (3 marks)

All oxygenation occurs within the placenta; therefore, blood passing back from the placenta needs to pass directly into the left side of the circulation. This is achieved in two ways. First, the ductus venous is present within the liver to direct blood into the right atrium of the heart. Second, the foramen ovale shunts oxygenated blood from the right atrium into the left atrium.   (3 marks)

Fetal blood

The first fetal blood cells are formed on the surface of the yolk sac and haemopoiesis continues at this site until the third month. During the fifth week of life, the extramedullary haemopoiesis begins in the liver and, finally, bone marrow production starts at 7–8 weeks and reaches its peak by the 26th week of life.   (3 marks)

Haemoglobin F (HbF) is the most common in the fetus. HbF has a higher affinity for oxygen than adult haemoglobin (HbA), therefore enhancing gaseous exchange across the placenta. The production of HbA is initiated at around 28 weeks and, by term, it makes up 20 per cent of the blood haemoglobin.   (3 marks)

See Chapter 6, *Obstetrics by Ten Teachers*, 18th edition.

Antenatal care

5 Write short notes on booking blood investigations, antenatal visit examination and customized antenatal care.

Blood tests

All pregnant women should be encouraged to undergo screening for a number of health issues. The following blood tests are normally performed. A full blood count is taken to screen for anaemia and thrombocytopenia. The woman's blood group and red-cell antibodies are also determined. If the woman is rhesus negative, then she will be offered prophylactic anti-D administration at 28 and 32 weeks' gestation. Maternal blood will be screened for hepatitis B, human immunodeficiency virus (HIV) and syphilis. If any of these are positive, then appropriate treatment is initiated. In the case of HIV, this includes commencing antiviral drugs and offering Caesarean section. If the patient was a carrier or had presence of a recent infection, then the fetus should be actively and passively immunized at birth. Syphilis is treated with high-dose maternal antibiotics.   (5 marks)

Antenatal visit examination

At each visit, the mother's blood pressure is tested to screen for pre-eclampsia. The maternal abdomen is palpated to confirm fetal presentation. The symphysis–fundal height is measured to screen fetal growth.   (5 marks)

Customized antenatal care

Through the process of booking and antenatal care it may become apparent that a women and her pregnancy have risk factors that are not met by standard services. In these cases, referral to other caregivers may be appropriate to ensure that the woman has customized antenatal care. One example of this is diabetes, where women receive customized care within a dedicated clinic.   (5 marks)

See Chapter 7, *Obstetrics by Ten Teachers*, 18th edition.

Antenatal imaging and fetal assessment

6 Describe the use of ultrasound in obstetrics.

Ultrasound scanning is one of the most commonly used modalities in obstetrics. It can be carried out throughout all gestations to assess the fetus and surrounding structures.   (1 mark)

In the first trimester, it is used to confirm viability, for accurate dating, and the diagnosis of twin pregnancies. It is also used for the determination of chorionicity in twin pregnancies. Uterine abnormalities and ovarian cysts may be determined during the first trimester scan. Within the first trimester, there is opportunity for ultrasound screening with the nuchal translucency.   (4 marks)

During the second trimester, the anomaly scan is performed. This is undertaken at approximately 20 weeks. It involves a detailed structural survey of the fetus to detect any abnormalities. Uterine artery Doppler scans may be performed to determine if the mother has an increased risk of developing pre-eclampsia. Cervical length may also be determined and utilized to assess the risk of preterm labour. Monochorionic twins may be assessed for signs of twin–twin transfusion.   (5 marks)

During the third trimester, ultrasound can be utilized to determine the placental site accurately. However, the most important role of ultrasound during the third trimester is that of determining fetal well-being. This is achieved by the measurement of fetal growth parameters, liquor volume and umbilical artery Doppler measurements.   (4 marks)

See Chapter 8, *Obstetrics by Ten Teachers*, 18th edition.

Prenatal diagnosis

7 Describe the techniques used for invasive prenatal diagnosis.

Amniocentesis is the most commonly used diagnostic test and can be performed from 15 weeks to term. It is carried out on pregnancies that have been identified as high risk by prior screening or history.   (2 marks)

Amniocentesis is performed with a trans-abdominal needle and carries fetal loss rates of 0.5–1.5 per cent.   (2 marks)

Chorionic villus sampling (CVS) is an alterative to amniocentesis. It has the similar indication of increased risk by prior screening. However, it has the advantage that it can be performed either transabdominally of transvaginally from 10 weeks' gestation to term.   (2 marks)

Chorionic villus sampling has a similar fetal loss rate to that of amniocentesis. One of the major disadvantages of CVS is the potential for contamination of the sample by maternal cells or the presence of placental mosaicism; this can lead to either a false-negative result, or make the result difficult to interpret.   (2 marks)

Cordocentesis is the final method of invasive fetal testing. This involves the direct sampling of fetal blood from the umbilical vein. The test is usually performed at or after 20 weeks' gestation.   (2 marks)

See Chapter 9, *Obstetrics by Ten Teachers*, 18th edition.

Second trimester miscarriage

8 Define second trimester miscarriage and outline the possible aetiologies.
Second trimester miscarriage is defined a pregnancy loss occurring between 12 and 24 weeks' gestation.
(1 mark)

The likely aetiologies behind second trimester losses vary with gestation. At 12–15 weeks, the predominant cause will be the same as first trimester losses: fetal chromosomal and structural anomalies. (2 marks)

A specific iatrogenic risk factor for late miscarriage is mid-trimester amniocentesis. This is usually performed at between 16 and 18 weeks' gestation and carries a risk of miscarriage of 1 in 200. (2 marks)

At the end of the second trimester, between 19 and 23 weeks, the commonest factors underlying miscarriage will be those linked to premature labour. Overdistension of the uterus, either by multiple pregnancy or polyhydramnios, leads to increased myometrial contractility and premature shortening and opening of the cervix. (4 marks)

Intrauterine bleeding irritates the uterus, leading to contractions, membrane damage and early rupture.
(1 mark)

Ascending infection from the vagina may pass through the cervix and reach the fetal membranes. This may have the effect of stimulating prostaglandin release and trigger contraction of the uterus. (2 marks)

Cervical weakness that has occurred as a result of previous surgical injury or a congenital defect may allow the cervix to shorten and open prematurely, the membranes then prolapse and may be damaged by stretching or direct contact with a bacterial pathogen. (2 marks)

See Chapter 10, *Obstetrics by Ten Teachers*, 18th edition.

Antenatal obstetric complications

9 A 26-year-old woman presents in clinic at 30 weeks' gestation. The community midwife has referred her because she is 'large for dates'. An ultrasound scan has demonstrated polyhydramnios. Discuss the possible causes of polyhydramnios in this pregnancy.
The causes of polyhydramnios can be divided into maternal, fetal and placental. The aim of any investigation of polyhydramnios is to establish a diagnosis, so that a prognosis can be determined. (2 marks)

Initially a full maternal history should be taken. This should include past medical history, as there are various diseases that can cause fetal polyhydramnios. The most common maternal disease associated with polyhydramnios is poorly controlled diabetes mellitus. Therefore, a random blood glucose level should be obtained and this should be followed by an oral glucose tolerance test, if indicated. Maternal red cell antibodies should be checked to exclude isoimmunization, as this is associated with fetal hydrops. (4 marks)

A detailed ultrasound should be arranged to check fetal growth, quantify the amniotic fluid index and examine for fetal abnormality. (1 mark)

Fetal abnormalities that can cause polyhydramnios include the following.
- Neuromuscular conditions that have the effect of obstructing the swallowing of amniotic fluid by the fetus.
- Fetal gastrointestinal abnormalities, including oesophageal and duodenal atresia. These block the ingestions of liquor into the fetus.
- Fetal hydrops, which should be excluded on an ultrasound scan, as this is associated with polyhydramnios secondary to cardiac failure or anaemia.
- Twin-to-twin transfusion is a rare cause of acute polyhydramnios in the recipient sac of monochorionic twins. It is associated with oligohydramnios in the other sac and requires urgent treatment by amniodrainage.

A detailed examination of the placenta may reveal a chorioangioma. (5 marks)

See Chapter 11, *Obstetrics by Ten Teachers*, 18th edition.

Twins and higher order multiple gestations

10 Outline the complications that may occur with a twin pregnancy.
Complications that occur in twins can be divided into those that occur in all twins and those that occur specifically to monochorionic twins. Monochorionic twins have specific complications owing to the fact that both twins share the same placenta. (2 marks)

The overall perinatal mortality rate for twins is six times higher than for singletons. The main contributing factor to this high rate is preterm delivery. (2 marks)

Spontaneous preterm delivery is an ever-present risk in any twin pregnancy and approximately half of all twin pregnancies deliver prematurely. In a dichorionic pregnancy, the chance of late miscarriage is approximately 2 per cent, and for monochorionic twins the risk is as high as 12 per cent. (2 marks)

Compared to singleton pregnancies, the risk of poor growth is higher in each individual twin alone and substantially raised in the pregnancy as a whole. In dichorionic twins, each fetus runs twice the risk of a low birth weight and there is a 20 per cent chance that at least one twin will suffer poor growth. The chance of poor fetal growth for monochorionic twins is almost double that for dichorionic twins. (3 marks)

Compared to singleton pregnancies, twins carry at least twice the risk of a baby with a birth defect. Each dichorionic twin pregnancy has at least twice the risk of a structural anomaly. In contrast, monochorionic twins carry a risk that is four times higher. (2 marks)

Chromosomal abnormality risk increases with maternal age independent of the number of fetuses. Therefore, in monozygotic twins, the risk is the same as for maternal age as both fetuses arise from the same egg. However, dizygotic twins have twice the risk, as the fetuses come from two different eggs. (2 marks)

All monochronic twins share vascular anastomoses and it is an imbalance in the blood flow across these anastomoses that causes the specific complication of twin-twin transfusion syndrome. (1 mark)

See Chapter 12, *Obstetrics by Ten Teachers*, 18th edition.

Disorders of placentation

11 A 24-year-old woman presents at 36 weeks in her first pregnancy. She has a blood pressure of 140/100 mmHg and urine dipstix shows 3+ proteinuria. Outline the management of this woman.
The most likely diagnosis is pre-eclampsia; however, this needs to be confirmed. A full history is required to ascertain whether there are any risk factors for pre-eclampsia. These include a family history of pre-eclampsia and multiple pregnancy. (2marks)

She should be admitted for both maternal and fetal assessment. Maternal assessment should include a full blood count to determine platelet count. Urea and electrolytes should be determined to assess renal function. Liver function tests should also be performed. A 24-hour urine collection should be initiated to confirm that the urinary protein is greater than 0.3 g/save. An urgent mid-stream urine and microscopy should be sent to exclude a urinary tract infection. (3 marks)

A full medical examination of the woman should be undertaken, including; a neurological examination of reflexes, which are brisk in pre-eclampsia. An abdominal palpation will demonstrate whether the fetus is clinically small for dates. (3 marks)

Cardiotocography (CTG) should be performed to assess immediate fetal well-being. If there are any abnormalities noted, then delivery should be considered. An ultrasound scan is useful to determine fetal well-being and presentation. (2 marks)

A diagnosis of pre-eclampsia should merit delivery. A vaginal examination should be performed to assess the cervix for favourability for induction of labour. If the cervix is unfavourable, then induction with prostaglandin pessaries is indicated. If an artificial rupture of the membranes is possible, then this should be undertaken. The fetus should be monitored continuously throughout labour. This woman requires close observation with regard to blood pressure and urine output, and one-to-one midwifery care. (3 marks)

See Chapter 13, *Obstetrics by Ten Teachers*, 18th edition.

Preterm labour

12 A 27-year-old woman, who is 30 weeks' gestation in her first pregnancy, is admitted from home with a history of painful contractions. Outline the management of this problem.
The likely differential diagnosis from the scenario is that of either preterm labour with or without membrane rupture. (1 mark)

The first step is to take the relevant history. This should determine whether there are any risk factors for either preterm labour or preterm rupture of the membranes (PROM). The common risk factors for both PROM and preterm labour that should be enquired about are twin pregnancy, uterine abnormalities, cervical damage (cone biopsy or repeat dilatation). It should also be determined whether there is a history of recurrent antepartum haemorrhage or sepsis. A full social history should be taken to determine whether the women smokes or takes drugs, and her social class, as all these factors increase the risk of preterm labour. (4 marks)

The diagnosis of preterm labour is difficult as women often present with vague cramp like pains and discomfort. The coexistence of bleeding should always be taken seriously. An increased analgesia requirement can also help refine the diagnosis. The most reliable diagnostic feature of PROM from the history is that of a sudden rush of fluid per vaginum. (3 marks)

A full examination should be undertaken. Abdominal palpation may reveal the presence of uterine tenderness, suggesting abruption or chorioamnionitis. Infection may lead to an increased pulse and temperature. A careful speculum examination should be performed to determine if there is any pooling of liquor and a visual assessment of cervical dilation is possible. (2 marks)

Maternal well-being should be assessed with measurement of blood pressure, pulse and temperature. A full blood count should be performed to determine if there is an increase in the white cell count indicating infection. While the speculum examination is being undertaken, a high vaginal swab (HVS), a fibronectin and a nitrazine test can be performed. A positive fibronectin test increases the probability of preterm delivery. Similarly a positive nitrazine test increases the probability of PROM. (3 marks)

Fetal assessment should include CTG to determine if there is a fetal tachycardia indicative of infection. An ultrasound scan can yield important information on liquor volume and cervical length can be determined if PROM has been excluded. (2 marks)

Maternal steroids should be given to induce fetal lung maturity. Tocolysis should be considered to allow the administration of maternal steroids. If PROM has been confirmed, then a 10-day course of erythromycin should be commenced, as this has been shown to improve neonatal outcome. If the HVS is positive for beta-haemolytic streptococcus, then intravenous antibiotics should be administered during labour. If labour continues, then continuous fetal monitoring should be initiated. (3 marks)

See Chapter 14, *Obstetrics by Ten Teachers*, 18th edition.

Medical diseases of pregnancy

13 A 24-year-old woman with poorly controlled insulin-dependent diabetes attends a general practitioner (GP) clinic, she is planning to start a family. Outline the advice specific to her condition that you would give regarding pregnancy.

She should be advised that poor glucose control in pregnancy increases the risk of congenital anomalies and also increases the risk of miscarriage. However, with good control, these risks are substantially reduced. (2 marks)

She should be advised that she will require hospital care and that this will take the form of a joint clinic with an obstetrician, diabetic physician, diabetic nurses and dieticians. (2 marks)

The aim of treatment is to maintain the blood glucose levels as near normal as possible. Insulin requirements go up during pregnancy and these will require careful monitoring. She should monitor her own blood glucose levels and have blood taken for haemoglobin A1c to monitor long-term control. She is at increased risk of both diabetic ketoacidosis and hypoglycaemia, and should be educated about the signs and symptoms of both. (3 marks)

It should be explained that an ultrasound scan at approximately 20 weeks' gestation would examine for structural anomalies especially cardiac and neural tube defects. (2 marks)

There is also a risk that both diabetic nephropathy and retinopathy will worsen with pregnancy; however, these complications usually improve postdelivery. There is an increased risk of pre-eclampsia, which will require regular monitoring of blood pressure and urine. (2 marks)

There is also an increased risk of polyhydramnios, which is associated with an increase in premature delivery. Poor control is associated with macrosomia and an increased rate of shoulder dystocia. The unexplained stillbirth rate is increased after 36 weeks and careful fetal monitoring will be necessary. (4 marks)

During labour, normoglycaemia should be maintained using a sliding scale of insulin and blood glucose should be tested hourly. Continuous fetal monitoring will be required during labour in view of the increased risk of her pregnancy. (2 marks)

See Chapter 15, *Obstetrics by Ten Teachers*, 18th edition.

Perinatal infections

14 Write short notes on HIV, parvovirus and beta-haemolytic streptococcus.

HIV

This is caused by a RNA retrovirus. There is no indication that pregnancy causes the progression of the disease in the mother. There is no evidence that pregnancy increases the risk of progression from HIV to the acquired immunodeficiency syndrome (AIDS). (3 marks)

HIV has been shown to have specific effects on the pregnancy; there is an increased risk of miscarriage, preterm delivery and intrauterine growth restriction. (3 marks)

Vertical transmission occurs in 25–40 per cent of pregnancies where there is no intervention. It is thought that the majority of transmission occurs around the time of delivery and subsequent breast feeding. Three interventions have been shown to reduce the vertical transmission rate: avoiding breast feeding, elective Caesarean section, and antiviral medication during the later half of pregnancy and into the neonatal period. (4 marks)

Parvovirus

Parvovirus B19 is the cause slap cheek syndrome in children. The infection is asymptomatic in 50 per cent of children and 25 per cent of adults. (2 marks)

In approximately 15 per cent of infections occurring during pregnancy, the fetus becomes chronically infected. This leads to a persistent anaemia *in utero*, which may develop into non-immune hydrops. This may resolve spontaneously or may require a blood transfusion. (3 marks)

The diagnosis of primary parvovirus is confirmed by demonstration of virus-specific IgM in the maternal serum. If this is demonstrated within the maternal serum, then the fetus needs close monitoring for signs of hydrops. However, parvovirus is not a teratogenic virus. (3 marks)

Beta-haemolytic streptococcus

This is an asymptomatic bacterial commensal of the gut and genital tract. It is carried asymptomatically in approximately 20–40 per cent of women. (2 marks)

It may cause severe neonatal infection and death. Although it can be detected on vaginal culture, screening and treatment are not beneficial because of frequent recolonization post-treatment. (2 marks)

Therefore, the recommendation is that the organism should be sought by culture in complicated pregnancies or where there has been a previous preterm delivery. If the organism is present or has been shown to be present in a previous pregnancy, then intravenous antibiotics should be administered during labour. (2 marks)

The infants at most risk are premature, those with prolonged rupture of membranes and growth-restricted fetuses. (2 marks)

See Chapter 16, *Obstetrics by Ten Teachers*, 18th edition.

Labour

15 Define primary dysfunctional labour, and outline its causes and possible treatments.
Primary dysfunctional labour is defined as poor progress, less than 1 cm per hour, in the active phase of labour. (1 mark)

The progress of labour depends on three interconnected variables: the powers, the passages and the passenger. (2 marks)

The most common cause of poor progress is ineffective uterine action, which is more common in the primiparous women. The treatment modalities that are available are rehydration, artificial rupture of the fetal membranes and intravenous oxytocin. (2 marks)

For adequate progress in labour, the tight application of the presenting part to the cervix is vital. Therefore, any malpresentations of the passenger, such as a brow or breech presentation, may ultimately result in slow progress. (2 marks)

Cephalopelvic disproportion (CPD) is also a cause of primary dysfunctional labour, and implies anatomical disproportion between the fetal head and the pelvis. It can be due to a large head, a small pelvis or a combination of both. It should be suspected if labour progresses slowly despite oxytocin, the fetal head fails to engage, vaginal examination shows severe moulding and caput, and the head is poorly applied to the cervix. Oxytocin may overcome the relative CPD of an abnormal presentation, such as brow, but Caesarean section may the only recourse, if the fetus in a favourable position. (3 marks)

Although abnormalities of the bony pelvis may cause delay of labour, abnormalities of the uterus and the cervix may have a similar effect. An unsuspected lower uterine fibroid can prevent delay in descent of the fetal head and result in Caesarean section. Cervical dystocia, owing to a scarred non-compliant cervix, can also result in a similar outcome. (3 marks)

See Chapter 17, *Obstetrics by Ten Teachers*, 18th edition.

Operative interventions in obstetrics

16 Write short notes on ventouse and forceps

Ventouse

This is an instrument that utilizes suction to aid the delivery of the fetus. It can be used for both maternal and fetal indications. The main maternal indication is exhaustion after prolonged pushing in the second stage, but is may also be used when shorting of the second stage is an advantage, such with maternal cardiac disease. The main fetal indication is suspected fetal compromise in the second stage. (4 marks)

The contraindications to its use are face presentation, gestation less than 34 weeks and marked bleeding from a fetal blood sample site. The prerequisites for delivery with the ventouse are fully dilated, station below the ischial spines, position known, good contractions, maternal bladder empty, adequate analgesia and maternal cooperation. (6 marks)

The commonest maternal complication is genital tract trauma. The main fetal complications are cephalhaematoma and, rarely, serious intracranial injuries. (2 marks)

Forceps

Obstetric forceps can be divided into two distinct groups: non-rotational or rotational forceps. (2 marks)

Non-rotational forceps have similar maternal and fetal indications to the ventouse. Non-rotational forceps have both a cephalic and a pelvic curve. Although the general indications for forceps and ventouse are similar, there are several specific indications for forceps: face presentation, bleeding from a fetal blood sample, the aftercoming head of a breech presentation, and delivery prior to 34 completed weeks. Obstetric forceps can also be utilized to aid delivery of the fetal head at Caesarean section. (6 marks)

Kjelland's (rotational) forceps lack the pelvic curve and this allows their rotation within the pelvis. The rotational forceps have additional indications for malpresentations, such as an occipital posterior position or deep transverse arrest. (2 marks)

The commonest maternal complication is maternal trauma. The forceps are less likely to cause cephalhaematoma but may cause rare, serious, intracranial injuries. (2 marks)

See Chapter 18, *Obstetrics by Ten Teachers*, 18th edition.

Obstetric emergencies

17 Write short notes on cord prolapse, shoulder dystocia and primary postpartum haemorrhage.

Cord prolapse

This is defined as a loop or loops of umbilical cord that fall through the cervix in front of the presenting part. Cord prolapse is associated with prematurity and malpresentations. This occurs in approximately 1 in 500 deliveries. (2 marks)

The diagnosis is usually made on vaginal examination because of an abnormal CTG. If the cord is through the vulva, it should be replaced to keep it warm. Urgent Caesarean section is required unless the cervix is fully dilated and assisted delivery can be performed safely. (4 marks)

While the Caesarean section is being arranged, it is vital that the umbilical vein is reduced to allow oxygen to pass to the fetus. This is achieved by placing the mother on all fours in a 'head down' position. A hand should be placed in the vagina to push the presenting part up. (2 marks)

Outcome depends on many factors including gestation and other pregnancy complications. . (2 marks)

Shoulder dystocia

This is defined as difficulty in delivery of the fetal shoulder. The incidence varies between 0.2 and 1.2 per cent of deliveries. (2 marks)

There are several risk factors that predispose to shoulder dystocia. These are: large fetus, small mother, maternal obesity, diabetes mellitus, prolonged first stage of labour, prolonged second stage of labour and assisted vaginal delivery. (2 marks)

Shoulder dystocia should be managed by a sequence of manoeuvres designed to facilitate delivery without fetal damage. The initial response to a shoulder dystocia should be a call for senior help. Excess traction should be avoided at all times. The legs should be hyperflexed and abducted at the hips. Suprapubic pressure should be applied to adduct the fetal shoulders. This should overcome >85 per cent of shoulder dystocia. If this fails, then more complex manoeuvres are required. These involve internal rotation of the fetal shoulders and delivery of the posterior arm. (4 marks)

Following delivery, the mother and her partner need to be debriefed regarding the events surrounding the delivery. (2 marks)

Postpartum haemorrhage

This is defined as excess blood loss (>500 mL) after delivery. This can be further subdivided into primary (within the first 24 hours) and secondary (up to 6 weeks) postpartum haemorrhage. (2 marks)

The most common cause of massive blood loss is uterine atony. This accounts for 90 per cent of cases. The first step is to stop the bleeding, which can be initially achieved by uterine massage or bimanual compression. Uterine contraction can then be maintained by pharmacological methods; these include the use of ergometrine and high-dose Syntocinon. The bladder should be emptied to aid contraction. If the uterus still fails to respond, then prostaglandin F2-alpha can be administered systemically or directly into the myometrium. (4 marks)

However, if the bleeding continues despite adequate uterine contraction, the next most common cause is genital tract trauma. The patient will require an examination under anaesthesia to explore the genital tract and repair the damage sustained. (2 marks)

If bleeding still persists, then clotting should be checked urgently as disseminated vascular coagulation may be present and needs to be corrected with blood products. (2 marks)

See Chapter 19, *Obstetrics by Ten Teachers*, 18th edition.

The puerperium

18 A 26-year-old woman who is 8 days postdelivery following a normal delivery is admitted with a pyrexia of 38.5°C. Discuss the possible diagnosis, investigations and treatments.

Postpartum pyrexia is a common occurrence, with an incidence of approximately 5 per cent. The aetiology can be broadly divided into three separate categories: infection of the urogenital tract; breast engorgement/infective mastalgia; and distant infection. (3 marks)

The most common cause of postnatal pyrexia is a urinary tract infection. The patient will present with dysuria, frequency and lower abdominal pain. This pain will be localized over the bladder and may radiate to the loins. A clean catch urine specimen should be collected and dipstix analysis may show protein and nitrates. The specimen should be sent for microscopy and culture. A full blood count, and urea and electrolytes should be sent as a general investigation of all women with pyrexia. Antibiotic therapy should be initiated; however, this should be altered depending on the results of urine culture. (5 marks)

Endometritis is another common infection that occur in the postnatal period. It presents with fever, rigors and an associated offensive vaginal discharge. A vaginal swab should be taken and antibiotics commenced. (3 marks)

Breast engorgement/infective mastalgia will present with a history of breast pain. Examination may reveal an enlarged erythematous breast. Anti-inflammatory drugs can be used to alleviate the pain and antibiotics, if infection is considered. If a breast abscess is present, it will need incision and drainage. (4 marks)

Chest infections are another cause of pyrexia that needs to be excluded, especially in a patient with an underlying chest problem, such as asthma. The patient may present with a productive cough. Examination would reveal evidence of consolidation at the lung bases. Sputum should be sent for culture. Antibiotics and supportive therapy with oxygen and physiotherapy are required. (3 marks)

Deep vein thrombosis may present as a postpartum pyrexia. The patient may complain of a painful swollen leg and calf tenderness. Examination would reveal an enlarged calf that would be red, swollen and hot to the touch. A duplex Doppler of the leg would confirm the diagnosis. Anticoagulant treatment should be initiated. (3 marks)

A pulmonary embolism may also present with pyrexia and, therefore, any patient where the diagnosis is questioned should be investigated. This may necessitate a ventilation/perfusion (V/Q) scan, and treatment with anticoagulants. (2 marks)

See Chapter 20, *Obstetrics by Ten Teachers*, 18th edition.

Psychiatric disorders in pregnancy and the puerperium

19 Discuss the possible psychiatric sequelae of pregnancy and how they might be treated.
Disturbances in the emotional state are common in the postnatal period. Up to 80 per cent of women will experience some form of emotional alteration. It most commonly occurs between days 3 and 10. (2 marks)

Mild postnatal depression affects 7 per cent of postnatal women. It is associated with social adversity, single status and poor support. The history is of an insidious onset of insomnia and difficultly in coping. The most effective treatment for mild depression is counselling, which in this group is as effective as antidepressant therapy. (4 marks)

Severe postnatal depression occurs in 3–5 per cent of all women. Most cases can be detected at the 6-week postnatal check by use of the Edinburgh postnatal score. A total of 30 per cent of those women with this condition will present within the first 3 months after delivery. They may present with a history of early morning wakening, altered appetite and ahedonism. The management should include explanation and reassurance. Tricyclic antidepressant therapy is effective with results observed within 2 weeks of commencing treatment. The course should be maintained for 6 months. (4 marks)

Postpartum psychosis affects 2 in 1000 women. One-third of these women will present will an acute episode of mania, while the other two-thirds will present with depression. Acute management should be aimed at sedation with neuropleptic drugs, which allows both containment and assessment. (3 marks)

A psychiatrist with an interest in postpartum psychiatric disorders should perform an assessment and it should coincide with admission to the nearest mother and baby unit. The patient should be continued on an oral neuroleptic agent, such as haloperidol. However, these drugs have extrapyramidal side effects, which can be treated with procyclidine. Lithium carbonate can be used for the mother who presents with a manic pathology. For women with severe depression, the firstline treatment is electroconvulsive therapy. The mother should be continued on treatment for at least 6 months and advised that there is a 50 per cent recurrence rate. (3 marks)

See Chapter 21, *Obstetrics by Ten Teachers*, 18th edition.

Objective structured clinical examination questions

1 Maternal and perinatal mortality: the confidential enquiry

Perinatal mortality is used as a measure of antenatal care.
a) Define perinatal mortality.
b) List three of the main causes of perinatal mortality.
c) Name two drugs that may have contributed to the fall in the perinatal mortality rate.
d) List the classification systems used by the Confidential Enquiry into Maternal and Child Health (CEMACH).

2 Conception, implantation and embryology

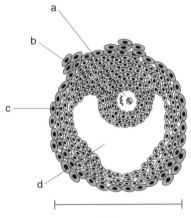

20 mm
Pre-ovulatory follicle

Figure 4.1 Adapted from Baker PN (ed) *Obstetrics By Ten Teachers*, 18th edition. London: Edward Arnold 2006.

a) Name the four structures labelled a, b, c and d.
b) Describe the process of meiosis.
c) Describe how pregnancy can be diagnosed and how it can be confirmed to be intrauterine.

3 Physiological changes in pregnancy

A 25-year-old woman in her first pregnancy attends a booking clinic at 12 weeks' gestation.
a) Describe the cardiovascular changes that have occurred.
b) Outline the physiological function and changes that have occurred in human chorionic gonadotrophin (hCG).
c) This woman goes on to have a normal vaginal delivery at term. She opts to breast feed the baby. Outline the physiological changes that occur within the mother with breast feeding.

4 Normal fetal development

A 22-year-old is admitted to the labour ward at 27 weeks pregnant. She is complaining of regular painful tightening. She describes having a mucus show the previous night, but denies any history of preterm rupture of membranes. On examination, she is distressed and requiring analgesia. Vaginal examination reveals that she is fully dilated with bulging forewaters. She delivers a live female infant that weighs 800 g.
a) Describe the physiological changes that occur in the cardiovascular circulation with birth.
b) Describe the physiological changes that occur in the respiratory system with birth.
c) What are the four main risks to the baby of premature delivery and how can these be minimized?

5 Antenatal care

A 30-year-old woman attends a routine booking clinic.
a) Take a booking history.
b) Explain the tests and scans that she will have during pregnancy assuming she has no risk factors.

6 Antenatal imaging and fetal assessment

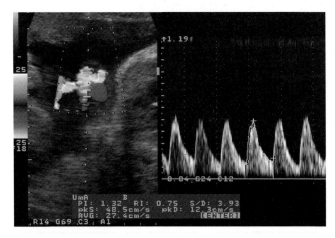

Figure 4.2

a) What is this investigation?
b) What is this picture showing?
c) What is RI?
d) What waveforms are abnormal?
e) What does it predict?

7 Prenatal diagnosis

A couple arrive in your antenatal clinic. They are both known to be carriers of the common mutation of the cystic fibrosis.
a) What are their chances of having a baby affected by cystic fibrosis?
b) What is the commonest mutation of the gene?
c) How can the diagnosis be made prenatally?
d) How early may the prenatal diagnostic test be made?

8 Second trimester miscarriage

Miss M is a 22-year-old single parent. She has had two previous miscarriages from two different partners. Her last pregnancy ended in a miscarriage at 18 weeks after being admitted with backache. She is now 22 weeks pregnant by her dating scan. She has been admitted to the labour ward with low back pain and a mucus loss.
a) What is the likely diagnosis?
b) What are the key points in the examination and investigation?
c) Miss M then starts to have painful regular contractions. How would you manage her labour?

9 Antenatal obstetric complications

The community midwife refers a 25-year-old woman in her second pregnancy to an antenatal clinic: clinically examination has shown the fetus to be in the breech position. An ultrasound scan confirms an extended breech presentation. You are asked to counsel this woman as to the possible options that are available for her management.

10 Twins and higher-order multiple gestations

A 32-year-old woman attends your booking clinic. She has just had a dating scan that confirms the presence of twins. The ultrasound report demonstrates that these are monochorionic diamniotic twins.
a) Define monozygotic twins.
b) Describe how chorionicity is determined by ultrasound scan.
c) Outline the risk of multiple pregnancy.
d) Outline the specific risks of monochorionic twins?

11 Disorders of placentation

An 18-year-old in her first pregnancy is admitted to the antenatal ward for observation. She is 26 weeks pregnant. Consider the following blood results:

Blood test	24 weeks	26 weeks
Serum urate (μmol/L)	150	230
24-hour urinary protein (g/save)	0.6	3.5
Platelet count	230	120

a) What is the most likely diagnosis?
b) List three maternal signs that would help guide our management.
c) What are three possible maternal complications of this disease if its remains untreated?
d) What investigations would you perform on the fetus?
e) How should this woman by managed?

12 Preterm labour

A 26-year-old Caucasian woman presented at 25 weeks' gestation in her first pregnancy. She gives a good history of ruptured membranes 3 hours prior to admission. On clinical examination, no uterine activity was noted. The maternal blood pressure was 140/75 mmHg, the temperature was 37°C and the pulse rate was 80 beats per minute. An aseptic speculum examination revealed clear fluid in the vagina.

a) Outline four investigations that would be useful in the further management of this patient with confirmed ruptured fetal membranes.

b) At what gestational age can a fetus survive outside the womb?

c) With regard to women delivering after preterm rupture of the fetal membranes, what postnatal complications are important?

d) How would you advise this woman in her next pregnancy?

13 Medical diseases of pregnancy

Mrs MV is known to have pre-existing cardiac disease.

a) What is the most common acquired cardiac lesion?

b) What are the effects of cardiac disease on pregnancy?

c) How should her labour be managed?

14 Perinatal infections

A 35-year-old woman comes to a booking clinic. She has had a routine human immunodeficiency virus (HIV) test at her booking visit; this has shown her to be HIV positive. She has been counselled regarding the diagnosis of HIV.

a) What type of virus is HIV?

b) Name two types of cell that have CD4 receptors.

c) Outline two strategies of treatment that are available.

d) What interventions have been shown to reduce the transmission of HIV to the baby?

15 Labour

You are asked to examine the following chart.

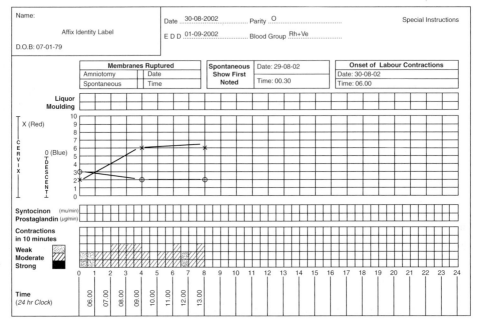

Figure 4.3

a) What is the chart called?
b) Describe the chart in front of you.
c) Describe the stages of labour.
d) What does abnormal labour pattern does the diagram illustrate?
e) How would you manage this obstetric problem?

16 Operative interventions in obstetrics

The following illustration shows an instrument that will be seen on any labour ward.

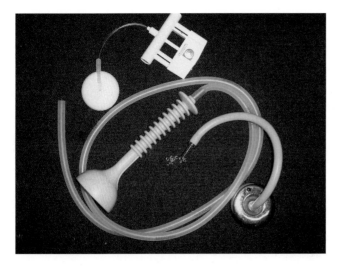

Figure 4.4

a) Name the instrument in the picture.
b) Give three indications for its use.
c) Give three situations were this instrument is contraindicated.
d) Give two maternal complications of this instrument.
e) What are the possible fetal complications of this instrument?

17 Obstetric emergencies

Mrs Smith has delivered a 3500 g baby on the delivery suite, where she was given intramuscular syntometrine. However, she has continued to lose blood and the estimate is 1000 mL. She is not clinically shocked and you are to see her because of her blood loss.
a) Define postpartum haemorrhage.
b) List the action you would take once you arrived to see this woman.
c) List the four most common causes of postpartum haemorrhage.

18 The puerperium

You are asked to see a 37-year-old woman in labour ward. She had an emergency Caesarean section for breech presentation 8 days ago. Over the last few hours, she has become breathless and has developed chest pain.
a) What is the most likely diagnosis?
b) What in the history would you ask to aid your diagnosis?
c) What would you look for on examination?
d) What investigations would you carry out to confirm the diagnosis?
e) What are the treatment options that are available?

19 Psychiatric disorders in pregnancy and the puerperium

A 27-year-old mother is seen by the community midwife 5 weeks after having a Caesarean section for failure to progress in the first stage of labour. She describes being miserable and starts to cry.
a) What is the mostly likely diagnosis?
b) What other symptoms might she have?
c) How is this condition treated?
d) Name a psychiatric disorder specific to pregnancy.
e) Outline the treatments that are available.

20 Neonatology

a) List three different deliveries where a trained neonatal resuscitator should be present.
b) Describe the Apgar score and how it is used.
c) Describe how you would manage a neonate that has been delivered without respiratory effort, but with a heart rate of >100 beats per minute and is centrally cyanosed.
d) Describe level 2 neonatal intensive care.

OSCE answers

1 Maternal and perinatal mortality: the confidential enquiry

a) Perinatal mortality rate is defined as the number of stillbirths and early neonatal deaths per 1000 live births and stillbirths.

b) Any three of the following: congenital anomaly; severe immaturity; infection; intracranial haemorrhage; isoimmunization; and unknown.

c) Maternal steroids and surfactant.

d) The extended Wriggleworth, the obstetric (Aberdeen) classification, and the fetal and neonatal factor classification.

See Chapter 3, *Obstetrics by Ten Teachers*, 18th edition.

2 Conception, implantation and embryology

a) 1, Oocyte; 2, zona pellucida; 3, granulosa cells; 4, follicular fluid.

b) Meiosis begins with diploid cells. The cell then undergoes an initial cell division that leads to two haploid daughter cells. During the second division, no DNA replication occurs. Thus, 23 double-stranded chromosomes will separate into single-stranded chromosomes to form the nucleus of each daughter cell.

c) The first sign of pregnancy is a missed period and can be confirmed by several methods. The pregnancy test measures the hormone human chorionic gonadotrophin (hCG) and commercial available kits are sensitive to 25 IU/L in urine. Quantitative serum hCG assay levels greater than 15 IU /L will usually denote a pregnancy. Ultrasound is commonly used to detect pregnancy. Transvaginal ultrasound will demonstrate a gestation sac 4–5 weeks after the last menstrual period and a fetal heart between 5 and 6 weeks. Abdominal ultrasound will demonstrate a gestation sac between 5 and 6 weeks, and a fetal heart a week later.

See Chapter 4, *Obstetrics by Ten Teachers*, 18th edition.

3 Physiological changes in pregnancy

a) Pregnancy is associated with dramatic cardiovascular changes, which occur from an early gestation. Overall there is a 10–20 per cent increase in the maternal heart rate and a 10 per cent increase in the stroke volume. These increases the cardiac output by 30–50 per cent. Associated with these changes are decreases in the maternal mean arterial pressure and in the peripheral vascular resistance.

b) Human chorionic gonadotrophin is composed of α and β subunits. hCG levels increase dramatically over the first 10 weeks. After 10 weeks, hCG reduces in concentration until 12 weeks, when it plateaus for the remainder of pregnancy. During early pregnancy, hCG has a major role in maintaining the function of the corpus luteum and the production of progesterone.

c) The serum prolactin concentrations increases throughout pregnancy. However, it does not promote lactation during this time, as its function is antagonized by oestrogen. The rapid fall in oestrogen within the first 48 hours after birth allow lactation to occur. Early sucking promotes lactation by increasing the posterior pituitary release of oxytocin and prolactin. Oxytocin causes the myoepithelial cells to contract and express milk, and prolactin to increase milk synthesis.

See Chapter 5, *Obstetrics by Ten Teachers*, 18th edition.

4 Normal fetal development

a) At birth, the cardiovascular system undergoes extensive remodelling under the changed haemodynamics of the now activated pulmonary system. In addition, the cessation of the umbilical blood flow in the ductus venosus causes a fall in the right atrial pressure and closure of the foramen ovale. Ventilation of the lungs opens the pulmonary circulation, with a rapid fall in the pulmonary vasculature resistance. The ductus arteriosus closes functionally within a few days of birth.

b) The fluid within the lung is reabsorbed. Compression of the chest at delivery forces out approximately one-third of the fluid and the release of adrenalin promotes reasorption of the rest. Surfactant is released, triggered by adrenalin and steroids. There is a fall in the capillary pressure of the lungs that occurs with the expansion of the alveoli, and the vasodilatory effect of oxygen. Respiratory movements of the chest commence.

c) Respiratory distress syndrome may lead to hypoxia. The administration of antenatal steroids to the mother reduces the risk and severity. In this case, antenatal steroids were not administered; however, the severity of respiratory distress syndrome can be reduced by the administration of surfactant. Hypothermia is a common problem related to the large surface area, lack of subcutaneous fat and keratinized skin. This large surface area also predisposes to dehydration. This can be reduced by nursing the infant in an incubator. Jaundice secondary to liver immaturity is common in the preterm infant; this can be treated with phototherapy. Periventricular haemorrhage and intraventricular haemorrhage commonly lead to cerebral palsy.

See Chapter 6, *Obstetrics by Ten Teachers*, 18th edition.

5 Antenatal care

a) The booking history should include the following: name; age; occupation; past obstetric history; past medical history; treatment history; and social history.

b) This question is best approached by dividing it into tests that are performed during the various trimesters of pregnancy.

First trimester

All pregnant women are encouraged to undergo screening for a number of health issues, which may have an impact on the pregnancy or the fetus. The following tests are performed routinely during the first trimesters:

- A full blood count is used to screen for anaemia and thrombocytopenia, both of which may require further investigation.
- Maternal blood group is determined, which will help with cross-matching at a later date. Rhesus status will be determined and prophylaxis will be offered at 28 and 34 weeks, if the mother is rhesus negative.
- Rubella status will be determined as vertical transmission carries serious risk of congenital abnormalities, especially in the first trimester. Women who are found to be non-immune should be advised to avoid infectious contacts.
- Hepatitis B status should be determined, so that passive and active immunization can be offered to the baby postdelivery.
- All women should be offered human immunodeficiency virus (HIV) testing as the use of antiretroviral agents, elective Caesarean section and avoidance of breast-feeding reduces the vertical transmission to less than 5 per cent.
- A dating ultrasound would be offered to all women. This has the benefits of accurate dating.

Second trimester

During the second trimester, at around 15 weeks, the triple test would be offered to all pregnant women. This is used to indicate the risk of the mother having a baby with Down's syndrome.

Third trimester

Measurement of blood pressure occurs at all antenatal visits; however, its main role is during the late second and early third trimester as a screening test for pre-eclampsia. Urine will also be analysed at all antenatal visits for protein, blood and glucose. This is used to detect infection, pre-eclampsia and gestational diabetes.

See Chapter 7, *Obstetrics by Ten Teachers*, 18th edition.

6 Antenatal imaging and fetal assessment

a) This is an umbilical artery Doppler.
b) The picture shows a normal umbilical artery Doppler waveform.
c) Resistive index; this is calculated from the maximum umbilical artery systolic velocity − the minimum umbilical end-diastolic velocity/the maximum umbilical artery systolic velocity. When this value rises above the 95th centile of the range, this implies that the fetal placental perfusion is faulty.
d) Absent or reversed end-diastolic flow.
e) Absent or reversed end-diastolic flow have been shown to correlate strongly with fetal distress and intrauterine death.

See Chapter 8, *Obstetrics by Ten Teachers*, 18th edition.

7 Prenatal diagnosis

a) This is an autosomal recessive disorder. Therefore, if both parents are carriers, then the chances of having an effected child are 1:4 in each pregnancy.
b) The commonest mutation is the delta 508 mutation and this is present is 68 per cent of cases.
c) This could be diagnosed parentally from a chorionic villus biopsy.
d) The chorionic villus biopsy can be performed at any time after 10 weeks' gestation.

See Chapter 9, *Obstetrics by Ten Teachers*, 18th edition.

8 Second trimester miscarriage

a) The combination of two previous losses that presented with backache would suggest mid-trimester loss.
b) A general examination should be performed to check that the woman is well. This should include the patient's vital signs: pulse, temperature and blood pressure. A temperature may suggest infection, as would a tachycardia. Abdominal examination should be performed to palpate for contractions. Fetal heart auscultation should be performed to confirm fetal viability. Initially, a sterile speculum examination should be performed and a vaginal swab taken. Visualization of the cervix will determine whether it is dilating.

   A cervico-vaginal swab should be obtained to exclude infection. A urine sample should be obtained to exclude urinary tract infection, which may precipitate uterine activity. A full blood count should be taken to look for signs of infection. An ultrasound scan should be performed to confirm viability and gestation.
c) Adequate analgesia is essential so the patient suffers as little distress as possible. Vaginal delivery will almost always occur due to the small size of the fetus. Some of these babies will show signs of life and the parents need to be warned of this to avoid unnecessary distress. The parents should be offered contact details of support groups.

See Chapter 10, *Obstetrics by Ten Teachers*, 18th edition.

9 Antenatal obstetric complications

There are three available management options that need to be discussed with the patient. These are: elective Caesarean section; external cephalic version (ECV); and vaginal breech delivery. The candidate would be expected to take a brief obstetric history. This would be to determine if there were any factors in the history that would be a contraindication to vaginal breech delivery or ECV.

The term breech trial demonstrated that there was a reduction in the perinatal mortality and morbidity with elective Caesarean section over vaginal breech delivery. However, there are some factors that would increase the strength of recommendation for a Caesarean section, these being a large or small baby, a small pelvis on pelvimetry, previous Caesarean section and an extended fetal neck.

External cephalic version is carried out between 36 and 37 weeks' gestation. The procedure has been shown to reduce the number of Caesarean sections due to breech presentation. Contraindications to ECV are placenta praevia, oligohydramnios, previous Caesarean section, multiple gestation and pre-eclampsia. The risks of the procedure, which need to be outlined, are placental abruption, premature rupture of the fetal membranes, cord accident, transplacental haemorrhage and fetal bradycardia.

Vaginal breech delivery is still an acceptable option, if the mother understands the increased risks to the fetus. There are a number of factors that increase the likelihood of a successful breech delivery: normal size baby, flexed neck, multiparous, breech deeply engaged, and positive mental attitude of the woman.

See Chapter 11, *Obstetrics by Ten Teachers*, 18th edition.

10 Twins and higher-order multiple gestations

a) Monozygotic twins arise from a single fertilized ovum that splits into two identical structures. The type of monozygotic twins depends on how long after conception this splitting occurs.

b) The most reliable time to determine chorionicity is at the end of the first trimester. In dichorionic twins, there is a extension of the placental tissue into the base of the intertwin membrane, this is known as the 'lambda' sign. In monochorionic twins, this sign is absent and the membrane joins the uterine wall in a 'T'-shape.

c) There is an increased risk of intrauterine growth restriction compared to singleton pregnancies. The risk of fetal anomaly is greater in all twin pregnancies; however the risk is highest in monochorionic twin pregnancies. There is an increased risk of preterm labour in all twin pregnancies. The overall perinatal mortality rate for twins is six times higher than for singleton pregnancies.

d) Monochorionic twins carry a risk of twin-to-twin transfusion syndrome. This occurs due to vascular anastomoses between the two fetoplacental circulations. This is a potential dangerous complication, which, without treatment, will lead to miscarriage or severe preterm delivery in 90 per cent of cases.

See Chapter 12, *Obstetrics by Ten Teachers*, 18th edition.

11 Disorders of placentation

a) The most likely diagnosis based on the blood picture is pre-eclampsia.

b) Any three of the following: blood pressure >140/90 mmHg; hyperreflexia; clonus; papilloedema; visual disturbances; small for gestational age.

c) Three of the following: eclampsia; cerebrovascular accidents; renal failure; adult respiratory distress syndrome.

d) An ultrasound scan for fetal growth and liquor volume. Umbilical artery Doppler scans should be performed.

e) Treat blood pressure with antihypertensives. Administer steroids to accelerate lung maturity. Monitor fetus and indices, and consider delivery with worsening indices. Inform the neonatal unit about impeding delivery.

See Chapter 13, *Obstetrics by Ten Teachers*, 18th edition.

12 Preterm labour

a) The first investigation that should be initiated is genital tract swabs. This may guide antibiotic therapy, if required. An ultrasound can give valuable information on the amniotic fluid volume. There is a direct correlation between the amount of amniotic fluid and the time to labour. Maternal well-being should be regularly assessed; this should include pulse and blood pressure, and some advocate serial C-reactive protein and white cell count. Fetal well-being should also be regularly monitored with cardiotocography.

b) Neonatal survival can rarely occur at 23 weeks, is possible between 24 and 25 weeks, and is likely after 26 weeks.

c) Any woman delivering after preterm rupture of the fetal membranes is at increased risk of endometritis and postpartum haemorrhage. Therefore, prophylactic antibiotics should be considered.

d) This woman should be advised that there are non-modifiable and modifiable risk factors, and that she is at 20 per cent risk of preterm birth in this pregnancy in view of her previous history. Smoking is an independent risk factor and cessation of smoking will reduce her risk of preterm labour. Drug abuse is also linked to preterm labour and can be stopped. An interpregnancy interval of less than 1 year is associated with an increased risk and, therefore, delaying subsequent pregnancies may reduce the risk. An early dating scan should be arranged to ensure precise assessment of fetal gestational age. Vaginal swabs should be taken and tested for bacterial vaginosis (BV) and Group B streptococcus. Treatment of women with BV in high-risk populations has been shown to reduce the preterm birth rate by 60 per cent.

See Chapter 14, *Obstetrics by Ten Teachers*, 18th edition.

13 Medical diseases of pregnancy

a) Mitral stenosis.

b) Prematurity is a common effect of cardiac disease. This can be either iatrogenic or because the fetus is small for gestational age. There is also an increase in the maternal mortality; however, this varies depending on the cardiac lesion. There is also a 5 per cent risk that the fetus will have a congenital heart defect.

c) Induction of labour should be avoided unless for obstetric indications. Prophylactic antibiotics should be given to prevent bacterial endocarditis. A close monitoring of fluid balance should be initiated. Anaesthesia should be discussed with a senior anaesthetist. The second stage of labour should be kept short.

See Chapter 15, *Obstetrics by Ten Teachers*, 18th edition.

14 Perinatal infections

a) HIV is an single-stranded retrovirus that binds to CD4 receptors.

b) T-helper lymphocyctes, macrophages, dendritic cells and microglia cells present CD4 receptors.

c) There are two main strategies used in the treatment of HIV. If there is no evidence of immunodeficiency, then antiretoviral drug therapy is commenced as highly active retroviral therapy. This is a combination of several drugs that include nucleoside reverse transcriptase inhibitors, a non-nucleoside reverse transcriptase inhibitor and a protease inhibitor. If there is evidence of immunodeficiency, then treatment is aimed at prevention of opportunistic infection.

d) Vertical transmission occurs in 25–40 per cent of pregnancies, if there are no interventions to reduce the risk. The three intervention that have been shown to reduce the vertical transmission of HIV are: avoiding breast feeding, elective Caesarean section, and the use of antiviral drugs in the later half of pregnancy and neonatal period.

See Chapter 16, *Obstetrics by Ten Teachers*, 18th edition.

15 Labour

a) The chart is a partogram of X.

b) This is a partogram. It is a pictorial presentation of the process of labour.

c) The first stage of labour is defined as the time from the diagnosis of labour to full dilatation of the cervix. The second stage of labour is defined as the time from full dilation of the cervix to the delivery of the fetus or fetuses. The third stage of labour is defined as the time from the delivery of the fetus to delivery of the placenta.

d) Secondary arrest of labour due to irregular uterine contractions.

e) From the partogram, the membranes are still intact, as there is no liquor draining. Therefore, an artificial rupture of the membranes should be performed, then the patient should be examined 2 hours after this. If there is still no progress, then syntocinon should be commenced.

See Chapter 17, *Obstetrics by Ten Teachers*, 18th edition.

16 Operative interventions in obstetrics

a) Ventouse.

b) Delay in the second stage, fetal distress in the second stage and maternal conditions requiring a short second stage.

c) Face presentation, gestation less than 34 weeks and marked active bleeding from the fetal blood sample site.

d) Vaginal lacerations and cervical injury.

e) Chignon, cephalohaematoma, neonatal jaundice and lacerations of the fetal scalp.

See Chapter 18, *Obstetrics by Ten Teachers*, 18th edition.

17 Obstetric emergencies

a) Postpartum haemorrhage is defined as excess blood loss (1000 mL) in the first 24 hours after delivery.

b) Call for help, massage the uterus, gain intravenous access, administer high-dose syntocinon, and determine the cause of the bleeding and deal with it.

c) This can be remembered with the simple 'four Ts': tonic uterus; trauma; tissue – check placenta complete; thrombin – clotting.

See Chapter 19, *Obstetrics by Ten Teachers*, 18th edition.

18 The puerperium

a) The mostly likely diagnosis in a woman presenting with this history is a pulmonary embolism.

b) The patient may complain of a cough and haemoptysis. She may also complain of a swollen, painful calf secondary to a deep venous thrombosis (DVT) of the leg. There may be a family history of DVT or pulmonary embolism (PE).

c) Examination may reveal tachypnoea, raised jugular venous pressure and right ventricular heave. The patient's calf may also be swollen and painful, suggesting a DVT.

d) A chest X-ray should be performed. This is usually normal; however, it excludes other causes of breathlessness. An electrocardiogram should be performed, but this may also be normal except for a sinus tachycardia. Arterial blood gases would show hypoxaemia and hypercapnia. The definitive test for a PE is a V/Q scan. This will demonstrate a ventilation/perfusion mismatch.

e) The initial treatment is with intravenous heparin or subcuticular low-molecular-weight heparin.

See Chapter 20, *Obstetrics by Ten Teachers*, 18th edition.

19 Psychiatric disorders in pregnancy and the puerperium

a) The mostly likely diagnosis is postpartum depression.

b) She may complain of early morning waking, a loss of appetite, low energy, lack of enjoyment, anxiety, thoughts of self-harm.

c) There are three main treatment options. These include remedy of social factors. However, several randomized trials have demonstrated the benefits of non-directive counselling from specially trained midwives and health visitors. If pharmacotherapy is deemed necessary, tricyclic antidepressants or selective serotonin reuptake inhibitors (SSRIs) are widely used. There is evidence to support their safety in the postnatal breast feeding women.

d) Puerperal psychosis.

e) The treatment is aimed at treating the acute psychotic event. This can be achieved with the use of neuroleptics, such a haloperidol or chlorpromazine. If there is a significant manic component to the presentation, then lithium carbonate should be initiated. Electroconvulsive therapy is an option in women with severe depressive psychosis. Antidepressants are used as a second-line therapy.

See Chapter 21, *Obstetrics by Ten Teachers*, 18th edition.

20 Neonatology

a) There are many circumstances were a trained resuscitator should be present. These include: preterm deliveries; vaginal breech delivery; significant fetal distress; serious fetal abnormality; rotational forceps; and Caesarean section.

b) The Apgar score is a tool that was developed to assist the recognition of an infant who is failing to make a successful transition to extrauterine life. It has five separate categories that are scored 0, 1 or 2, depending on the observation of the neonate to give a maximum of score of ten. The categories are appearance (central trunk colour), pulse rate, response to stimulus, muscle tone and respiratory effort. It should be recorded at 1 minute and 5 minutes unless there is a problem, when further observation should be recorded.

c) The baby should be dried and placed under a radiant heat source wrapped in a warm dry towel. The process of drying often provides enough stimuli to induce breathing. If there no response, then commence active resuscitation using five inflation breaths via a bag and mask, and summon help.

d) Level 2 intensive care is provided by specially trained nursing staff that care for two babies at a time. Examples would include babies requiring parenteral nutrition, having apnoeic attacks or requiring oxygen treatment, and weighing less than 1500 g.

See Chapter 22, *Obstetrics by Ten Teachers*, 18th edition.

Gynaecology

Extended matching questions

1 Embryology

A Mesonephric ducts
B Paramesonephric duct
C Mullerian system
D Sinovaginal bulbs
E Genital tubercle
F Genital folds
G Genital swellings
H Genital ridge

For each description below, choose the SINGLE most appropriate answer from the above list of options. Each option may be used once, more than once, or not at all.

1 Develop(s) into the lower portion of the vagina.
2 Form(s) the ovary.
3 Develop(s) into the labia minora.
4 Develop(s) into the labia majora.

2 Anatomy and physiology

A Aorta
B Internal iliac vein
C Renal vein
D Vena cava
E Superficial inguinal and femoral nodes
F Obturator, internal and external iliac nodes
G Paraaortic nodes
H External iliac vein

For each description below, choose the SINGLE most appropriate answer from the above list of options. Each option may be used once, more than once, or not at all.

1 Lymphatic drainage of the ovary.
2 Lymphatic drainage of the lower vagina and vulva.
3 Lymphatic drainage of the upper vagina and cervix.
4 Venous drainage from the left ovarian vein.

3 Normal and abnormal sexual development and puberty

A Cloacal cells
B 17-Hydroxyprogesterone
C Wolffian duct

D Testosterone
E Dihydrotestosterone
F Leydig cells

G SRY region
H Sertoli cells

For each description below, choose the SINGLE most appropriate answer from the above list of options. Each option may be used once, more than once, or not at all.

1 This is responsible for the production of TDF.
2 These cells are responsible for the production of Mullerian inhibitor.
3 These cells are responsible for the production of testosterone.
4 This is the hormone responsible for the development of the vas deferens, epididymis and seminal vesicles.

4 Disorders of the menstrual cycle

A Adenomyosis
B Stress incontinence
C Endometrial polyp

D Malignancy of the cervix
E Fibroids
F Pelvic inflammatory disease

G Endometrial malignancy
H Uterine prolapse

For each description below, choose the SINGLE most appropriate answer from the above list of options. Each option may be used once, more than once, or not at all.

1 Intermenstrual bleeding.
2 Postcoital bleeding.
3 Postmenopausal bleeding.
4 Painful periods.

5 Disorders of the menstrual cycle

Surgical treatments
A Transcervical resection
of the endometrium
B Vaginal hysterectomy

C Microwave ablation
D Endometrial curettage
E Manchester repair

F Myomectomy
G Abdominal hysterectomy
H Mirena

For each description below, choose the SINGLE most appropriate answer from the above list of options. Each option may be used once, more than once, or not at all.

1 A procedure for the investigation of menorrhagia but not a treatment.
2 An outpatient procedure that destroys the endometrium and fibroids up to 4 cm in diameter.
3 A procedure for women with fibroids who want to retain their fertility.
4 A definitive treatment for menorrhagia refractive to other treatments, if the uterus is not enlarged and ovarian conservation is required.

Medical treatments
A Cyclical progestogens
B Combined oral
contraceptive pill
C LNG-IUS

D Antifibrinolytics
E Antiprostaglandins
F Gonadotrophin-releasing
hormone analogues

G Danazol
H Gestrinone

For each description below, choose the SINGLE most appropriate answer from the above list of options. Each option may be used once, more than once, or not at all.

1 The 5-year prolonged exposure of the endometrium to progestogen to cause thinning of the endometrium and lighter menses.
2 This reduces production of prostaglandin E2 and reduces loss by up to 25 per cent.
3 This is to be taken from days 5 to 26 in anovulatory dysfunctional uterine bleeding; it regulates the cycle and promotes secretory endometrium in the second half of the cycle.
4 This promotes coagulation and reduces menstrual loss by 40 per cent.

6 Infertility

A Clomid
B Anovulation
C Oligospermia
D Azoospermia
E Polycystic ovary syndrome
F Chlamydia
G Androgen-secreting tumour
H Puregon

For each description below, choose the SINGLE most appropriate answer from the above list of options. Each option may be used once, more than once, or not at all.

1 This is associated with a raised free androgen index, low sex hormone-binding globulin and raised testosterone.
2 The commonest cause of tubal disease in the Western world.
3 The only treatment is donor insemination.
4 An oral treatment for anovulation.

7 Disorders of early pregnancy

A Threatened miscarriage
B Missed miscarriage
C Incomplete miscarriage
D Ectopic pregnancy
E Hydatidiform mole
F Heterotropic pregnancy
G Choriocarcinoma
H Septic miscarriage

For each description below, choose the SINGLE most appropriate answer from the above list of options. Each option may be used once, more than once, or not at all.

1 The proliferation of trophoblastic tissue with or without embryonic tissue.
2 The partial expulsion of products of conception with products of conception seen >65 mm in diameter on ultrasound scan.
3 Bleeding in pregnancy <24 weeks' gestation with fetal heart visible on ultrasound scan and closed cervical os.
4 Light bleeding, pelvic pain, shoulder tip pain, 6 weeks' gestation, empty uterus on ultrasound and fluid in pouch of Douglas.

8 Benign diseases of the cervix

A Squamous metaplasia
B Columnar epithelium
C Moderate dyskaryosis
D Severe dyskaryosis
E Borderline nuclear change
F Mild dyskaryosis
G Glandular atypia
H Arias–Stella change

For each description below, choose the SINGLE most appropriate answer from the above list of options. Each option may be used once, more than once, or not at all.

1 CIN1   2 CIN2   3 CIN3   4 CGIN

9 Benign diseases of the uterus

A Leiomyosarcoma
B Pedunculated leiomyoma
C Hyaline degeneration
D Adenomyosis
E Red degeneration
F Endometriosis
G Brenner's tumour
H Calcified degeneration

For each description below, choose the SINGLE most appropriate answer from the above list of options. Each option may be used once, more than once, or not at all.

1 This occurs as a result of disruption of blood supply (typically pregnancy-related).
2 Necrosis and cystic formation due to outgrowth of blood supply.
3 Fibroid change that is usually a postmenopausal manifestation.
4 Malignant change that accounts for less than 1 per cent of fibroids.

10 Endometriosis and adenomyosis

A Transcervical resection of the endometrium
B Laser ablation to endometrial deposits
C Hydrothermal ablation
D Total abdominal hysterectomy and bilateral salpingo-oophorectomy

E Medical therapy, such as the combined oral contraceptive pill
F Vaginal hysterectomy
G No treatment is indicated
H Surgical drainage and postoperative gonadotrophin-releasing hormone (GnRH) antagonist treatment

For each description below, choose the SINGLE most appropriate answer from the above list of options. Each option may be used once, more than once, or not at all.

1 Treatment for minimal endometriosis to improve chances of conception in patient with infertility.
2 Definitive treatment for Stage IV endometriosis, obliterated rectovaginal septum and bilateral endometriomata.
3 Asymptomatic endometriosis found on routine laparoscopy for sterilization.
4 Symptomatic endometriosis in a 23-year-old woman who wants children but is currently not contemplating pregnancy.

11 Benign diseases of the ovary

A A fibroma
B Serous cystadenoma
C A teratoma

D Endometroid tumour
E Clear cell tumour
F A granulosa cell tumour

G Brenner's tumour
H Mucinous cystadenoma

For each description below, choose the SINGLE most appropriate answer from the above list of options. Each option may be used once, more than once, or not at all.

1 A unilocular cyst with papillous processes usually occurring unilaterally.
2 A large unilateral multiloculated cyst lined by columnar epithelium and complicated with pseudomyxoma peritonii.
3 A large cyst usually containing unclotted blood with a ground-grass appearance on ultrasound.
4 This has a solid appearance with islands of transitional epithelium in dense fibrotic stroma.

12 Malignant disease of the uterus and cervix

A Subtotal abdominal hysterectomy
B Cold coagulation
C Wertheim's hysterectomy
D LLETZ (large loop excision of the transformation zone)

E Pelvic exenteration
F Bilateral salpingo-oophorectomy
G Palliative treatment
H Wertheim's hysterectomy and radiotherapy

For each description below, choose the SINGLE most appropriate answer from the above list of options. Each option may be used once, more than once, or not at all.

1 CIN2.
2 Ectopy.
3 Stage 1B cervical cancer.
4 Stage 2 cervical cancer.

13 Carcinoma of the ovary and Fallopian tube

A Laser laparoscopy
B Vaginal hysterectomy
C Total abdominal hysterectomy (TAH), bilateral salpingo-oophorectomy (BSO) and omentectomy
D Subtotal hysterectomy

E Unilateral salpingo-oophorectomy and peritoneal washings
F TCRE
G Wertheim's hysterectomy
H Debulking surgery and subsequent carboplatin or cisplatin/aclitaxel chemotherapy

For each description below, choose the SINGLE most appropriate answer from the above list of options. Each option may be used once, more than once, or not at all.

1 Stage 1B ovarian cancer.
2 Stage 3 epithelioid tumour.
3 Unilateral borderline tumour.
4 Endometriosis.

14 Infections in gynaecology

A Candida
B Chlamydia
C Bacterial vaginosis

D Trichomoniasis
E Herpes
F Syphilis

G Human immunodeficiency virus (HIV)
H Gonorrhoea

For each description below, choose the SINGLE most appropriate answer from the above list of options. Each option may be used once, more than once, or not at all.

1 A sexually transmitted disease typified by genital ulcers and painful vesicles.
2 A non-sexually transmitted infection typified by itchy sore vagina with a white 'curdy' discharge.
3 A non-sexually transmitted disease typified by an offensive fishy discharge.
4 A sexually transmitted disease typified by Gram-negative diplococci, and colonizing columnar and cuboidal epithelium; 50 per cent are found asymptomatically.

15 Urogynaecology

A Urodynamic stress incontinence
B Normal bladder function
C Poor detrusor contraction

D Bladder diverticulum
E Sensory urgency
F Urethral obstruction

G Detrusor overactivity
H Detrusor–sphincter dyssynergia

For each description below, choose the SINGLE most appropriate answer from the above list of options. Each option may be used once, more than once, or not at all.

1 Detrusor pressure rise >15 cm of water during filling associated with urgency.
2 A voiding detrusor pressure 10 cm of water and flow rate of 5 mL per second.
3 Leakage on coughing in the absence of detrusor contraction.
4 Voiding detrusor pressure >70 cm of water and peak flow rate 5 mL second.

16 Uterovaginal prolapse

A Anterior repair
B Shelf pessary
C Sacrospinous fixation
D Posterior repair
E Vaginal hysterectomy
F Sacrocolpopexy
G Ring pessary
H Manchester repair

For each description below, choose the SINGLE most appropriate answer from the above list of options. Each option may be used once, more than once, or not at all.

1 The treatment for vault prolapse in a frail elderly woman who would not be suitable for surgery.
2 The historical treatment for prolapse involving amputation of the cervical stump and plication of the uterosacral and cardinal ligaments.
3 The treatment of choice for a cystocele with no history of incontinence but poor voiding in a 50-year-old, sexually active woman.
4 Operation of choice for the treatment of vault prolapse in an elderly woman with multiple previous abdominal surgery who is not sexually active.

17 The menopause

A Tibolone
B Medroxyprogesterone acetate
C Transdermal patch containing 50 μg of oestrogen
D Norplant
E Conjugated equine oestrogen
F Echinacea
G Vagifem
H Implanon

For each description below, choose the SINGLE most appropriate answer from the above list of options. Each option may be used once, more than once, or not at all.

1 An oral hormone replacement therapy (HRT) preparation that is converted to oestrone by hepatic enzymes resulting in a plasma oestradiol (E2)/oestrone ration of 1:2.
2 A lipid-soluble preparation maintaining an E2/oestrone ratio of 2:1, which is similar to pre-menopausal physiological status.
3 A HRT with mild androgenic side effects, which may have a beneficial effect on low libido.
4 An essential part of HRT to reduce the risk of endometrial hyperplasia in women with a uterus.

18 Common gynaecological procedures and medico-legal aspects of gynaecology

Surgical complications
A TCRE
B Tension-free vaginal tape (TVT)
C Vaginal hysterectomy
D Posterior repair
E Cystoscopy
F Laparoscopy
G Abdominal hysterectomy for extensive endometriosis
H Flexible hysteroscopy

For each description below, choose the SINGLE most appropriate answer from the above list of options. Each option may be used once, more than once, or not at all.

1 Gas embolism.
2 Ureteric injury.
3 Damage to the bladder.
4 Uterine perforation.

EMQ answers

1 Embryology

1 D   2 H   3 F   4 G

The sinovaginal bulbs develop as outgrowths that canalize and form the lower portion of the vagina below the level of the hymen. The ovary is derived from three components: the genital ridge, underlying mesoderm and the primitive germ cells. The genital tubercle forms the clitoris, the genital folds the labia minora and genital swellings the labia majora.

See Chapter 2, *Gynaecology by Ten Teachers*, 18th edition.

2 Anatomy and physiology

1 G   2 E   3 F   4 C

Lymphatic drainage of the ovary is via a plexus of vessels lying in the infundibulopelvic folds to the para-aortic node on both sides of the midline. The lymphatic drainage of the lower third of the vagina follows that of the vulva to the superficial inguinal and femoral nodes, whilst the upper portion of the vagina follows that of the cervix to the obturator, internal and external iliac nodes. The venous drainage of the ovary is to the renal vein on the left and inferior vena cava on the right.

See Chapter 2, *Gynaecology by Ten Teachers*, 18th edition.

3 Normal and abnormal sexual development and puberty

1 G   2 H   3 F   4 D

The *SRY* gene lies on the short arm of the Y chromosome and is responsible for determination of testicular development as it produces TDF (testicular development factor). TDF stimulates the undifferentiated gonad to produce Mullerian inhibitor. The Leydig cells produce testosterone, which promotes development of the Wolffian ducts into the vas deferens, epididymis and seminal vesicles.

See Chapter 3, *Gynaecology by Ten Teachers*, 18th edition.

4 Disorders of the menstrual cycle

1 C   2 D   3 G   4 A

Abnormal bleeding outside the normal menstrual cycle should always be investigated. Intermenstrual bleeding is commonly associated with an endometrial polyp or luteal phase insufficiency. Postcoital bleeding should always be investigated by visualization of the cervix to exclude a cervical malignancy. Postmenopausal bleeding should be considered to be endometrial carcinoma until this has been excluded by either ultrasound and endometrial sampling, or hysteroscopy and curettage. Adenomyosis causes painful periods and is typified by a tender, bulky uterus.

See Chapter 4, *Gynaecology by Ten Teachers*, 18th edition.

5 Disorders of the menstrual cycle

Surgical treatments

1 D   2 C   3 F   4 B

An endometrial curettage is useful to gain histology of the endometrium and is often performed at the time of hysteroscopy. The endometrium can be either resected (transcervical resection of the endometrium; TCRE) or ablated using microwaves, hot water or a balloon filled with heated solutions. Any of these methods can result in reduced menstrual loss or amenorrhoea to various degrees. Myomectomy can be performed to remove large fibroids to allow symptomatic relief without removal of the uterus, thus retaining a woman's fertility. Pregnancy is contraindicated after (TCRE) or ablation. Hysterectomy is the definitive treatment for menorrhagia. The route is determined by the size of the uterus, the degree of uterine descent and the necessity for oopherectomy.

See Chapter 5, *Gynaecology by Ten Teachers*, 18th edition.

Medical treatments

1 C **2** E **3** A **4** D

The levonorgestrel intrauterine system (LNG-IUS) is an intrauterine device with a sleeve inpregnanted with slow-release levonorgestrel (progesterone). Prolonged exposure of the endometrium to progesterone causes thinning of the endometrium and reduces menstrual loss. Cyclical progesterone causes the endometrium to remain secretory until withdrawal of the progesterone, which results in menstruation. Antiprostaglandins, such as mefenamic acid, are non-steroidal anti-inflammatory drug (NSAID) derivatives and inhibit prostaglandin formation, whereas antifibrinolytics, such as tranexamic acid, inhibit lysis of formed clots. Both are useful in reducing loss in the regular cycle.

See Chapter 5, *Gynaecology by Ten Teachers*, 18th edition.

6 Infertility

1 E **2** F **3** D **4** A

Polycystic ovary syndrome is a condition associated with insulin resistance. Women are typically overweight, hirsute and have acne. The hormone profile of these women typically shows elevated androgens and a low sex hormone-binding globulin. Chlamydial infection is the commonest cause of pelvic inflammatory disease and tubal factor infertility in the West. Men suffering from azoospermia have no sperm to be harvested and hence can only have children either by adoption or donor insemination. Anovulation can be treated orally with Clomid or by intramuscular gonadotrophins (e.g. Puregon).

See Chapter 7, *Gynaecology by Ten Teachers*, 18th edition.

7 Disorders of early pregnancy

1 E **2** C **3** A **4** D

Molar pregnancies can be either partial or complete depending on whether embryonic tissue also develops. Incomplete miscarriage is associated with retained products of conception on ultrasound, whereas the uterus is empty after a complete miscarriage. If a viable pregnancy is confirmed on ultrasound after bleeding, it is defined as a threatened miscarriage. Ectopic pregnancies are typified by unilateral pain, blood in the pelvis, which causes diaphragmatic irritation and pain referred to the shoulder tip.

See Chapter 8, *Gynaecology by Ten Teachers*, 18th edition.

8 Benign diseases of the cervix

1 F **2** C **3** D **4** G

Dyskaryosis is a cytological diagnosis made on a cervical smear. Cervical intraepithelial neoplasia (CIN) is a histological diagnosis made on biopsy of cervical tissue. Mild dyskaryosis is analogous to CIN1, moderate dyskayosis to CIN2 and severe dyskaryosis to CIN3. Glandular atypia occurs in the columnar cells of the endocervical canal and is associated with Cervical glandular intra-epithelial neoplasia (CGIN) and adenocarcinoma.

See Chapter 9, *Gynaecology by Ten Teachers*, 18th edition.

9 Benign diseases of the uterus

1 E   2 C   3 H   4 A

Fibroids can undergo various forms of change. A sudden loss of blood supply causes pain and red degeneration typically seen in pregnancy. Slow outgrowth of its blood supply causes necrosis and cyst formation. After the menopause, fibroids may calcify. Rarely, leiomyosarcoma can develop from fibroids.

See Chapter 9, *Gynaecology by Ten Teachers*, 18th edition.

10 Endometriosis and adenomyosis

1 B   2 D   3 G   4 E

Endometriosis is a benign condition that has various treatments depending on the clinical situation. Asymptomatic endometriosis requires no treatment at all. The exogenous endometrial tissue is susceptible to endogenous oestrogen and the menstrual cycle. Mild to moderate endometriosis can be treated by administration of exogenous hormones, such as the combined oral contraceptive pill or GnRH agonists to downregulate the hypothalamic–pituitary–ovarian axis. Laser ablation to mild endometriosis has been shown to improve symptoms and improve chances of conception in women with subfertility. Once a woman's family is complete and there is extensive symptomatic disease, definitive treatment is necessary along with bilateral oophorectomy.

See Chapter 10, *Gynaecology by Ten Teachers*, 18th edition.

11 Benign diseases of the ovary

1 B   2 H   3 D   4 G

Ultrasound can be helpful in differentiating benign tumours. More often, histological classification is necessary to determine the origin and nature of the tumour.

See Chapter 11, *Gynaecology by Ten Teachers*, 18th edition.

12 Malignant disease of the uterus and cervix

1 D   2 B   3 C   4 H

Cervical ectopy is not a pre-malignant condition. It can be left alone, if it is asymptomatic in the presence of a normal smear and colposcopy. If it is symptomatic, then coagulation can be used. Preclinical disease that invades to a depth less than 3 mm and width of 7 mm can be safely treated with local excision (LLETZ). Treatment of clinical disease is usually with surgery, radiotherapy or both. If the disease is confined to the cervix, then surgery or radiotherapy can be used. Once it has spread outside the cervix, radiotherapy is the main treatment modality.

See Chapter 12, *Gynaecology by Ten Teachers*, 18th edition.

13 Carcinoma of the ovary and Fallopian tube

1 C   2 H   3 E   4 A

Stage 1b is confined to both ovaries with no ascites, or tumour on the external surface of the ovary and an intact capsule. In this case, TAH and BSO and omentectomy are sufficient. After Stage 1B, chemotherapy is also required. Unilateral borderline tumours can be treated by removing the affected ovary and taking peritoneal washings to check for spread. However, if the patient's family is complete and there is a suspicion of malignancy, TAH and BSO and omental biopsy may be more prudent. Endometriosis is a benign condition and can be ablated with a laser or diathermy.

See Chapter 13, *Gynaecology by Ten Teachers*, 18th edition.

14 Infections in gynaecology

1 E   2 A   3 C   4 H

Primary genital herpes is a sexually transmitted condition that presents with painful ulcers and vesicles, often with urinary retention due to pain. Candida is not sexually transmitted, and is a common condition presenting with a white discharge and red sore vagina compared with bacterial vaginosis, which has a typical 'fishy' odour and frothy discharge. Gonorrhoea and chlamydia are often asymptomatic. Chlamydia is the commonest cause of pelvic inflammatory disease (PID) in the West, but is diagnosed by enzyme-linked immunosorbent assay (ELISA), whereas gonorrhoea can be diagnosed on microscopy.

See Chapter 15, *Gynaecology by Ten Teachers*, 18th edition.

15 Urogynaecology

1 G   2 C   3 A   4 F

A rise in detrusor pressure associated with urgency is diagnostic of detrusor overactivity. Urodynamic stress incontinence is diagnosed in the absence of a detrusor contraction. A flow rate of 5 mL per second is reduced. In the presence of a high detrusor pressure, this would indicate a urethral obstruction. If the detrusor pressure was low and the flow rate also low, poor detrusor function would be more likely.

See Chapter 16, *Gynaecology by Ten Teachers*, 18th edition.

16 Uterovaginal prolapse

1 B   2 H   3 A   4 C

Surgery is unsuitable in frail women who could not tolerate general or regional anaesthesia, and so a pessary would be more appropriate. The Manchester repair is an operation that used to be performed for prolapse with an elongated cervix. It involved cervical amputation, anterior and posterior repair, and shortening the cardinal ligaments. Anterior repair is an effective treatment for cystocele but is not effective in treating stress incontinence. Abdominal surgery for vault prolapse (sacrocolpopexy) should be avoided if the patient is frail or has multiple previous abdominal procedures (concerns about adhesions). Sacrospinous fixation is a vaginal procedure for vault prolapse and has less morbidity associated.

See Chapter 17, *Gynaecology by Ten Teachers*, 18th edition.

17 The menopause

1 E   2 C   3 A   4 B

Hormone replacement therapy can be oestrogen alone in hysterectomized women, or oestrogen and progesterone in women with a uterus. Oestrogen can be taken orally and pass through the first-pass metabolism, or through transdermal patches, which will avoid hepatic enzymes. Tibolone has mild androgenic side effects and is useful in women with a low libido. Progesterone in various forms (e.g. medroxyprogesterone acetate) is necessary in women with a uterus to prevent endometrial hyperplasia.

See Chapter 18, *Gynaecology by Ten Teachers*, 18th edition.

18 Common gynaecological procedures and medico-legal aspects of gynaecology

1 F   2 G   3 B   4 A

Gas embolism can occur after laparoscopy, although it is rare. Women are usually consented about the risk of injury to the bowel or aorta from Veress needle insertion, trochar insertion and operative laparoscopy. Endometriosis can cause tethering of the ureter to the parametrium, thus increasing the risk of ureteric injury at hysterectomy. Bladder perforation is said to occur in 1–5 per cent of TVTs. Cystoscopy is routinely performed and, if recognized, the trochars can be removed and reinserted correctly and a draining catheter left for several days. Uterine perforation and even hysterectomy are possible at TCRE. This is reduced if rollerball or endometrial ablation is performed instead.

See Appendices 1 and 2, *Gynaecology by Ten Teachers*, 18th edition.

Chapter 6

Multiple choice questions

History and examination

1 With regard to clinical examination of the gynaecological patient:
a) Abdominal examination is mandatory as part of the gynaecological examination.
b) A chaperone is always needed for intimate examinations.
c) Palpation below a pelvic mass is possible.
d) Shifting dullness and fluid thrill can be seen due to urinary retention.
e) Bidigital examination can determine whether a pelvic mass is ovarian or uterine in origin.

Embryology, anatomy and physiology

2 The following statements apply to the human female pelvis:
a) The Fallopian tubes are lined by cilia to aid egg transport.
b) The middle portion of the Fallopian tube is called the ampulla.
c) The ovary is the only abdominal structure not covered by peritoneum.
d) The ovary is attached to the uterus by the round ligament.
e) The ovary has a central medulla of loose connective tissue and an outer cortex covered by cuboidal germinal epithelium.

3 Considering the bladder and rectum:
a) The bladder capacity is normally 700 mL.
b) The base of the bladder is closely related to the cervix and upper vagina, and can be damaged at hysterectomy.
c) The ureter passes in the broad ligament in its lower portion and curves beneath the uterine artery, along the lateral vaginal fornix before entering the trigone of the bladder.
d) In its upper portion the ureter lies anterior to the ovary.
e) The rectum is covered by peritoneum on its front and sides in the lower two-thirds.

Normal and abnormal sexual development and puberty

4 In the XY genotype:
a) Androgen insensitivity results in an XY genotype and female phenotype but with normal testes.
b) In 5-alpha-reductase deficiency, virilization of the cloaca fails to occur owing to the failure of the conversion of testosterone to 17-hydroxyprogesterone.
c) In androgen insensitivity, Mullerian ducts regress owing to the production of Mullerian inhibitory factor.
d) In androgen insensitivity, the Wolffian ducts regress owing to the absence of an androgen receptor.
e) In 5-alpha-reductase deficiency, the Mullerian ducts fail to regress owing to the lack of Mullerian inhibitory factor.

5 In an XX phenotype female:
a) Rokitansky's syndrome is associated with failure of development of the uterus, cervix and vagina.
b) Often the ovaries are present in patients with Rokitansky's syndrome.
c) A failure of fusion of the mesonephric ducts would cause an abnormality of the uterus and cervix, and is associated with a degree of reproductive failure.
d) In congenital adrenal hyperplasia, 21-hydroxylase deficiency prevents the production of 17-hydroxyprogesterone in the adrenal gland.
e) Virilization of the fetus can be secondary to drugs ingested by the mother.

The normal menstrual cycle

6 Within the follicular phase of the menstrual cycle:
a) The follicular phase is always 14 days long to allow development of the follicle.
b) Follicle-stimulating hormone (FSH) stimulates the granulosa cells to produce oestrogen.
c) Each cycle usually involves the development, growth and ovulation of a single follicle.
d) Follicles over 20 mm need to be drained with ultrasound guidance.
e) Oestrogen and inhibin have a positive feedback on the pituitary to release FSH and luteinizing hormone (LH).

7 In relation to ovulation:
a) LH induces thecal cells to produce oestrogen.
b) FSH induces a rise in LH receptors
c) Ovulation occurs 14 hours after the LH surge.
d) The release of an oocyte from the follicle requires a sperm to lyse the follicle membrane and results in ovulation.
e) Ovulation can be confirmed by measurement of LH on day 14.

8 Within the luteal phase of the menstrual cycle:
a) The predominant hormone in the luteal phase is progesterone.
b) The granulosa cells of the corpus luteum have a rich vascular supply and have a yellow pigment owing to accumulation of cholesterol.
c) The luteal phase varies in duration depending on the time taken to degenerate a corpus luteum.
d) The corpus luteum continues to degenerate in early pregnancy.
e) Low levels of oestrogen and progesterone are the best indicators of the perimenopause.

Disorders of the menstrual cycle

9 Definitions:
a) Polymenorrhoea is defined as prolonged increased menstrual flow.
b) Oligomenorrhoea is defined as menses occurring at a <21-day interval.
c) Hypermenorrhoea is defined as excessive regular menstrual loss.
d) Amenorrhoea is defined as absence of menstruation for more than 12 months.
e) Menorrhagia is defined as menses at intervals of >35 days.

10 Regarding the investigation of menorrhagia:
a) A full blood count is mandatory.
b) Thyroid function tests are mandatory.
c) A hysteroscopy and endometrial biopsy should be performed in women over the age of 25.
d) A pelvic ultrasound scan is only indicated if one is suspicious of a pelvic mass or fibroids.
e) A hormone profile including mid-luteal progesterone is essential to differentiate between ovulatory and non-ovulatory dysfunctional bleeding.

Fertility control

11 With regard to the progesterone-only pill:
a) The progesterone-only pill has a higher failure rate in women under the age of 40 than in women over the age of 40.
b) The progesterone-only pill has a lower risk of ectopic pregnancy.
c) The progesterone-only pill has a 3-hour window.
d) The progesterone-only pill has a better bleeding profile compared with the combined oral contraceptive pill
e) The progesterone-only pill has a quicker reversibility compared with the combined oral contraceptive pill.

12 Considering the depot injection and hormonal implants:
a) There are two types of depot injection. One contains medroxyprogesterone acetate 150 and lasts for 12 weeks, the other contains norethisterone 200 and lasts for 8 weeks.
b) The depot is licensed for 2 years only, otherwise there is an increased risk of reduced bone density and osteoporosis.
c) The depot can cause amenorrhoea but irregular bleeding is also a significant side effect
d) The Implanon implant involves five rods to be inserted in the upper arm and lasts for 5 years
e) With the Implanon implant, the return to ovulation after the implant is removed usually takes up to 1 year.

13 Concerning the intrauterine contraceptive device (IUCD):
a) Modern IUCDs can last for 5–10 years.
b) The levonorgestrel intrauterine system (Mirena) is licensed for 8 years.
c) Heavy bleeding can be a common side effect with the Mirena.
d) The risk of pelvic inflammatory disease is increased with IUCD use.
e) There is an increased risk of ectopic with IUCD use.

14 The combined oral contraceptive pill (COCP):
a) Inhibits ovulation.
b) Improves cycle control.
c) Has a 3-hour window.
d) Is relatively contraindicated in patients with acute/severe liver disease.
e) Has a risk of venous thromboembolism (VTE) of 15 per 100 000 in third-generation preparations.

Infertility

15 Considering successful conception:
a) The single most important factor affecting the chance of a couple conceiving is the age of the female partner.
b) The rates of conception rapidly decline after the age of 30.
c) Tubal infertility is the main cause of infertility in the Western world.
d) The chance of spontaneous conception in a young couple with no adverse fertility factors is 50 per cent per cycle.
e) 85 per cent of healthy women aged 25 years will conceive after 12 months.

16 With regard to the investigation of the infertile couple:
a) A full hormone profile, tubal patency testing and semen analysis should be completed on all couples attending a referral for primary infertility.
b) A mid-luteal progesterone >25 nmol/L confirms ovulation.
c) A semen analysis should be performed prior to laparoscopy and dye to test for tubal patency.
d) Hysterosalpingogram, and laparoscopy and dye insufflation will gain similar information and either can be used to assess tubal patency in all patients.
e) A single semen analysis with a volume of 1 mL, a concentration of 10 million/mL and 30 per cent reduced motility confirms oligospermia, and serum testosterone, gonadotrophins and prolactin analysis should be performed.

Disorders of early pregnancy

17 Concerning disorders of early pregnancy:
a) If the cervical os is open, it is a threatened miscarriage.
b) If transvaginal scan shows products of conception up to 20 mm in diameter, then surgical evacuation of the uterus is essential.
c) Serum β-hCG levels are useful in dating a pregnancy up to 12 weeks.
d) Ultrasound appearances of retained products of conception of <15 mm would be consistent with a complete miscarriage.
e) A snowstorm appearance on ultrasound is suggestive of choriocarcinoma.

18 With regard to miscarriage:
a) Total loss of conception after fertilization is around 50–70 per cent.
b) The total rate of clinical miscarriage is around one-quarter to one-third of all pregnancies.
c) Miscarriage is much greater before 6 weeks than after 9 weeks.
d) The rate of miscarriage is the same in women over 40 years of age compared with women under 40.
e) The most common cause of spontaneous miscarriage is infection.

19 In relation to molar pregnancy:
a) The uterus often appears larger on palpation than one would expect for gestation.
b) Hyperemesis is often seen in patients with molar pregnancies.
c) Ultrasound is not useful in the diagnosis of molar pregnancy and the diagnosis is usually made on histology.
d) Complete hydatidiform molar pregnancies have a diploid chromosomal constitution owing to duplication of paternal chromosomes and no maternal complement.
e) Partial molar pregnancies are usually diploid with duplication of the maternal set of chromosomes.

20 Considering ectopic pregnancy:
a) The rate of ectopic pregnancy is 0.5 per cent of all pregnancies.
b) Ectopic pregnancy is associated with Group B streptococcus infection.
c) Laparoscopic salpingectomy is the treatment of choice if the other tube is normal.
d) The rate of persistent trophoblast is increased if the patient has a laparoscopic salpingotomy rather than salpingectomy.
e) Methotrexate is contraindicated if the mass is >1 cm in diameter on ultrasound.

Benign diseases of the uterus and cervix

21 Indicate which of the following statements are true or false:
a) The transformation zone is an area of the cervix that marks the junction of the squamous epithelium of the ectocervix and vagina and the columnar epithelium binding the endocervix and the uterine cavity.
b) The situation of the transformation zone is affected by hormones and is easily visible at ovulation, pregnancy and in women using the combined oral contraceptive pill.
c) Outpouching of the columnar epithelium is termed as cervical erosion.
d) Columnar epithelium undergoes dysplasia to squamous epithelium under normal physiological conditions.
e) Vaginal discharge and postcoital bleeding seen in association with an ectopy can be initially treated with cold coagulation.

Benign diseases of the ovary

22 In dermoid cysts:
a) The malignancy rate is low (around 2 per cent).
b) 50 per cent are bilateral.
c) They are often lined by embryonic mesodermal structures.
d) Struma ovarii are dermoid tumours predominantly made of thyroid tissue.
e) Complications include torsion, chemical peritonitis and rupture.

23 In sex cord tumours:
a) All granulosa cell tumours are malignant, but are usually confined to the ovary and have a good prognosis.
b) Call–Exner bodies are pathognomonic of theca cell tumours.
c) Many theca cell tumours cause postmenopausal bleeding and endometrial carcinoma.
d) Meigs' syndrome is the combination of fibroma, ascites and pleural effusions.
e) Virilization is seen as 75 per cent of Sertoli–Leydig cell tumours.

24 The following factors on ultrasound are suspicious of malignancy:
a) A single loculated cyst of 7 cm diameter.
b) Multiple cysts around the periphery of the ovary with a dense stroma.
c) A single frond floating within a cyst.
d) Solid elements and septae.
e) Calcification and fats.

Malignant disease of the uterus and cervix

25 With regard to cervical cancer:
a) Cervical cancer is the third commonest cancer in women worldwide.
b) The incidence of cervical cancer has become far more common in young women since the 1980s.
c) The rate of deaths from cervical carcinoma has remained steady in recent years.
d) Human papillomavirus (HPV) types 14 and 18 are the most commonly associated with cervical cancer.
e) Cervical cancer is associated with previous infection with herpes simplex virus.

26 Concerning the cervical screening programme:
a) It is important when taking a smear that the squamocolumnar junction is identified and sampled.
b) Smears should be taken between the ages of 25 and 64.
c) Smears should be taken during pregnancy.
d) The screening programme screens for pre-malignant changes in the squamous and columnar epithelia
e) Mild dyskaryosis on smear is consistent with cervical intraepithelia or neoplasia (CIN1).

27 The following are risk factors for the development of cervical cancer:
a) HPV types 14, 17 and 31.
b) HPV types 16 and 18.
c) Family history of cervical cancer.
d) Smoking.
e) Previous chlamydial infection.

28 The following are risk factors for the development of endometrial cancer:
a) Obesity.
b) Diabetes.
c) Multiparity.
d) Early menopause.
e) Unopposed oestrogen therapy.

29 Considering treatments for cervical cancer:
a) Preclinical invasive disease that is a depth of 6 mm and a width of 7 mm can be treated by large loop excision of the transformation zone alone.
b) The risk of nodal involvement is 5 per cent if the depth of preclinical invasion is >3 mm.
c) A Wertheim's hysterectomy involves removal of the uterus, cervix, paracervical tissue, lymph node sampling and the upper two-thirds of the vagina.
d) At Wertheim's hysterectomy, the ovaries can be conserved.
e) One main complication of Wertheim's hysterectomy is poor bladder emptying owing to division of the S2,3,4 nerve roots of the pudendal nerve.

Carcinoma of the ovary and Fallopian tube

30 Regarding carcinoma of the ovary:
a) It is most common in developing countries.
b) The incidence is similar to carcinoma of the endometrium with similar prognosis.
c) The peak age is 80–90 years old.
d) The majority are epithelial in origin.
e) The mainstay of treatment is surgery and radiotherapy combined.

31 The following primary malignancies metastasize to ovary:

a) Lung.

b) Stomach.

c) Breast.

d) Thyroid.

e) Bone.

32 The following are risk factors for ovarian cancer:

a) Early menarche.

b) Early menopause.

c) Combined oral contraceptive pill usage.

d) Infertility.

e) Implanon implants.

33 In relation to ovarian cancer:

a) In the normal population, there is a lifetime risk of developing ovarian cancer of 5 per cent.

b) This usually applies to cystadenoma malignancy.

c) If a patient has one relative with ovarian cancer, their risk is increased to 10 per cent.

d) If a patient has two first-order affected relatives, their risk increases to 20 per cent.

e) *BRCA*1 or 2 gene-positive patients have a lifetime risk of ovarian cancer of 25 per cent.

34 The following are appropriate investigations for ovarian cancer:

a) Computerized tomography of the abdomen and pelvis.

b) Barium enema.

c) Intravenous pyelogram (IVP).

d) Ultrasound scan.

e) CA 125.

35 The following are common side effects of cisplatin use:

a) Peripheral neuropathy and hearing loss.

b) Hyperkalaemia.

c) Hypomagnesiumaemia.

d) Renal damage.

e) Visual disturbances.

36 The following are epithelial tumours:

a) Mucinous tumour.

b) Theca cell tumour.

c) Teratoma.

d) Brenner cell tumour.

e) Androblastoma.

37 Considering dysgerminomas:

a) The peak age is over the age of 45.

b) CA 125 is elevated in 50 per cent of cases.

c) They are mainly solid rather than cystic in nature.

d) They can cause a rise in alpha-fetoprotein and β-hCG.

e) Immature teratomas are benign and are commonly called dermoid tumours.

Conditions affecting the vulva and vagina

38 The following are causes of pruritis vulvae:
a) Lichen sclerosus.
b) Nephrotic syndrome.
c) Atrophy.
d) Vaginal discharge.
e) Diabetes.

39 The following apply to lichen sclerosis:
a) Sites commonly affected are the labia majora and mons pubis.
b) Labial adhesions.
c) White plaques.
d) It is commonly associated with autoimmune disorders such as diabetes and pernicious anaemia.
e) Areas of dark red–brown pigmentation.

Infections in gynaecology

40 The following are causes of benign vulval ulcers:
a) Tertiary syphilis.
b) Chancroid.
c) Herpes.
d) HPV infection.
e) Ulcerative colitis.

41 With regard to the lower genital tract:
a) The lower genital tract is lined by stratified squamous epithelium throughout life.
b) Vaginal pH is increased under the influence of oestrogen.
c) The pH after the menopause is around 7.0.
d) Candidal infection is increased in pregnancy, with combined oral contraceptive pill usage and broad-spectrum antibiotic usage.
e) Candida is the commonest cause of abnormal vaginal discharge in women of childbearing age.

42 Concerning herpes simplex virus:
a) The diagnosis is made on endocervical swabs.
b) Urinary retention and perineal pain are a common presentation.
c) Reactivation of the virus occurs after colonization of neurones in Onuf's nucleus.
d) Secondary infection in pregnancy necessitates delivery by lower segment Caesarean section.
e) Treatment with antiviral drugs is useful in established disease.

43 In relation to syphilis:
a) The causative organism is *Treponema pallidum.*
b) The TPHA is the most sensitive and specific test for syphilis.
c) Primary infection usually presents with a painful ulcer on the perineum.
d) Primary and secondary syphilis are not life threatening; however, tertiary neurosyphilis is life threatening, hence the importance of making the diagnosis.
e) Early treatment is with quadruple therapy of rifampicin, isoniazid, pyrazinamide and ethambutol.

Urogynaecology

44 Which of the following is true?

a) Stress incontinence is the diagnosis of involuntary loss of urine in association with a rise in intra-abdominal pressure in the absence of detrusor contraction.

b) Detrusor overactivity is the urodynamic observation of an involuntary increase in detrusor pressure during filling, which may be spontaneous but which may also be provoked by a cough. It is associated with urgency and occasional urge incontinence, frequency and nocturia.

c) Acute urinary tract infection or constipation can present as urinary incontinence in the elderly.

d) Urodynamic stress incontinence is usually ideopathic but, in a number of patients, may be caused by neuropathy, previous incontinence surgery and outflow obstruction.

e) Poor urinary stream is diagnostic of urethral obstruction.

Uterovaginal prolapse

45 Regarding the pathophysiology of pelvic organ prolapse:

a) Pelvic organ prolapse is commoner in nulliparous women than in multiparous women.

b) Pelvic organ prolapse is never seen in nulliparous women.

c) Prolapse is commoner after the menopause partly due to oestrogen deficiency.

d) Epidural in labour is a risk factor for the subsequent development of prolapse.

e) Forceps delivery is a risk factor for the development of prolapse.

The menopause

46 Within the human ovary:

a) The follicles are centrally placed in the medulla.

b) The cortex and medulla contain stroma of endodermal origin.

c) The stromal cells of the cortex and medulla produce predominantly androgens.

d) There is a decline in the number of primordial follicles from around 7 million at 6 months gestation to 1.5 million at birth.

e) Around 400–000 follicles that are present at puberty will progress to ovulation.

47 Considering the pathophysiology of the menopause:

a) Oestrogen is produced in the granulosa cells of the developing follicle.

b) Oestrogen is produced from the precursors of androstenedione and testosterone by the enzyme 17-hydroxylase.

c) Theca cells are stimulated by FSH and granulosa cells are stimulated by LH.

d) The first change in the endocrine system associated with the menopause is a fall in the hormone inhibin produced by the ovary.

e) Levels of FSH start to fall as a secondary effect in the menopause and thus prevent stimulation of the ovaries to produce oestrogen.

Common gynaecological procedures and medico-legal aspects of gynaecology

48 With regard to abdominal and vaginal hysterectomy.

a) Vaginal hysterectomy can only be performed if there is uterovaginal prolapse.

b) Abdominal hysterectomy is indicated if there is a suspicion of malignancy.

c) The recovery from a vaginal hysterectomy is slower compared to abdominal hysterectomy.

d) Recovery from a Pfannenstiel incision is quicker than from a midline incision.

e) The incidence of haematoma formation is greater after abdominal hysterectomy than after a vaginal hysterectomy.

49 **Which of the following statements are true?**
a) In induced abortion, the gestation is not to exceed 26 weeks.
b) The decision can be made by any registered doctor or medical practitioner as long as they are acting in good faith.
c) Pre-operative assessment of patients before termination includes a vaginal examination to date the pregnancy and, if there is any uncertainty about date, an ultrasound scan would be indicated.
d) The patient should have a chlamydia swab performed before theatre, as the incidence of chlamydia is higher in patients attending for termination of pregnancy.
e) A failed termination of pregnancy and continuation of the pregnancy is greater if termination is performed after 10 weeks.

MCQ answers

1 **True: a, b, e.** Shifting dullness and a fluid thrill are found with ascites or fluid within the peritoneal cavity.

See Chapter 1, *Gynaecology by Ten Teachers*, 18th edition.

2 **True: a, c, e.** The Fallopian tube has a lateral ampulla, middle isthmus and medial ostium. The ovary is attached to the cornua of the uterus by the ovarian ligament and to the hilum by the broad ligament.

See Chapter 2, *Gynaecology by Ten Teachers*, 18th edition.

3 **True: b, c.** The normal bladder capacity is 400 mL. The ureter lies lateral to the ovary passing through the ovarian fossa. The rectum is covered by peritoneum on the front and sides in its upper third, front in its middle third and not at all in its lower third.

See Chapter 2, *Gynaecology by Ten Teachers*, 18th edition.

4 **True: a, c, d.** 5-Alpha-reductase deficiency results in failure of virilization of the cloaca owing to the failure of conversion of testosterone to dihydrotestosterone. If this enzyme is absent, then the external genitalia will be female but the internal genitalia will be male. Mullerian ducts will regress as the testes still produce Mullerian inhibitory factor.

See Chapter 3, *Gynaecology by Ten Teachers*, 18th edition.

5 **True: a, b, e.** Failure of development of the paramesonephric ducts causes abnormalities in the uterus, cervix and is associated with a degree of reproductive failure. In congenital adrenal hyperplasia, 21-hydroxylase deficiency prevents the adrenal gland from producing cortisol. Failure of production of cortisol results via a feedback mechanism to stimulate the hypothalamus to produce increased adrenocorticotrophic hormone (ACTH), which in turn stimulates the adrenal gland to produce excessive amounts of the steroid precursor 17-hydroxyprogesterone. As a result, the adrenal gland produces excessive androgens, which lead to virilization of the cloaca.

See Chapter 3, *Gynaecology by Ten Teachers*, 18th edition.

6 **True: b, c.** The follicular phase varies in duration and this determines the cycle length (28–35 days). During each cycle, several primordial follicles develop, but only one follicle becomes dominant and continues to grow to around 20 mm in diameter. This follicle can be measured on ultrasound. It produces more oestrogen, while other follicles degenerate (undergo atresia). Ovarian cysts can grow up to 50 mm without any intervention necessary other than ultrasound observation. When cysts grow over 50 mm, there is a risk of ovarian torsion and, therefore, if they are persistent over 6 months observation, drainage or cystectomy are required. Oestrogen and inhibin have a negative feedback on the production of FSH.

See Chapter 4, *Gynaecology by Ten Teachers*, 18th edition.

7 **True: b.** Luteinizing hormone stimulates the thecal cells to produce progesterone. Ovulation occurs 24 hours after the LH surge. Ovulation is caused by the enzymatic degradation of the follicle membrane by endogenous plasminogen activators and prostaglandins. Fertilization involves the degradation of the zona pellucida of the oocyte by enzymes released from the acrosome of the sperm. Ovulation can be confirmed by measuring progesterone in the mid-luteal phase.

See Chapter 4, *Gynaecology by Ten Teachers*, 18th edition.

8 **True: a, b.** The luteal phase is always 14 days (i.e. progesterone peaks on day 21 of a 28-day cycle and day 28 of a 35-day cycle). If pregnancy occurs, serum beta-human chorionic gonadotrophin (sβ-hCG) is produced by the trophoblast. This has a similar structure to LH. Both LH and sβ-hCG cause the corpus luteum to mature (and not degenerate) in early pregnancy until the early placenta can produce progesterone, which is the predominant hormone of the luteal phase and early pregnancy. The granulosa cells have a yellow pigment called lutein, which is rich in cholesterol. Oestrogen and progesterone levels vary throughout the cycle. The perimenopause is associated with a high FSH. This blood test should be taken within 5 days of the last menstrual period, as this is when they should be at their lowest.

See Chapter 4, *Gynaecology by Ten Teachers*, 18th edition.

9 **True: c, d.** Polymenorrhoea is defined as menses occurring at a <21-day interval. Oligomenorrhoea is defined as menses at intervals of >35 days. Menorrhagia is defined as prolonged increased menstrual flow.

See Chapter 5, *Gynaecology by Ten Teachers*, 18th edition.

10 **True: a, d.** Thyroid function tests are only indicated if there is a clinical suspicion of thyroid disease. Royal College of Obstetricians and Gynaecologists (RCOG) guidelines suggest a hysteroscopy is indicated in women over the age of 40. If the cycle is regular, this is sufficient to suggest ovulation.

See Chapter 5, *Gynaecology by Ten Teachers*, 18th edition.

11 **True: a, c, e.** The progesterone-only pill has a higher risk of ectopic pregnancy compared with the combined oral contraceptive pill and has a worse bleeding profile compared to the combined pill. As it does not inhibit ovulation in all women, it is quicker to resume ovulation after stopping the progesterone-only pill, compared with the combined oral contraceptive.

See Chapter 6, *Gynaecology by Ten Teachers*, 18th edition.

12 **True: a, b, c.** The Implanon involves insertion of a single rod into the upper arm and this lasts for up to 3 years. The previous Norplant implants were licensed for 5 years and involved five rods into the upper arm but have since been withdrawn. The return to ovulation after removal of an Implanon implant is usually within 30 days.

See Chapter 6, *Gynaecology by Ten Teachers*, 18th edition.

13 **True: a, e.** The levonorgestrel intrauterine system (Mirena) is licensed currently for 5 years. Irregular heavy bleeding is a side effect associated with the copper coil; however, the Mirena is usually associated with reduction of menstrual loss. There is no increased risk of pelvic inflammatory disease with coil use; in fact, it is the same as with other contraceptive methods. The risk of infection is only increased at the time of insertion or removal.

See Chapter 6, *Gynaecology by Ten Teachers*, 18th edition.

14 **True: a, b.** The combined pill has a 12-hour window. Acute/severe liver disease is an absolute contraindication to COCP usage. The risk of VTE is 15 per 100 000 for second-generation users, 30 per 100 000 for third-generation users and 60 per 100 000 for pregnancy.

See Chapter 6, *Gynaecology by Ten Teachers*, 18th edition.

15 **True: a, e.** Rates of conception rapidly decline after the age of 35. Tubal infertility is the main cause of infertility in Africa; however, in the Western world, male factors or ovulation disorders are the most likely cause of infertility. A young couple with no adverse infertility factors have a 20 per cent chance of conceiving each cycle.

See Chapter 7, *Gynaecology by Ten Teachers*, 18th edition.

16 **True: c.** Investigations for infertility are expensive and some of them are invasive. Therefore, investigations should be directed towards each couple having gained an insight into the possible cause of infertility from the history. For example, a woman with a regular menstrual cycle need only require a mid-luteal progesterone to suggest ovulation occurs and does not need a full hormone profile. Further investigations are targeted according to the clinical picture. A low mid-luteal progesterone will confirm anovulation. A high progesterone of >30 nmol/L is certainly suggestive of ovulation but does not confirm ovulation. Ovulation can only be truly confirmed by serial scanning of ovarian follicles. However, in day to day use, a regular cycle and a progesterone level of >30 nmol/L is usually seen as indicative of ovulation.

Full investigations for ovulatory disorders and male factor infertility are mandatory prior to embarking upon laparoscopy and tubal patency testing, as this procedure does have a morbidity associated with it. A hysterosalpingogram will gain information on tubal patency and uterine cavity outline; however, this does not give any indication of pelvic disease, such as previous pelvic infection or endometriosis. Laparoscopy allows both the tubal patency to be assessed as well as staging degree of endometriosis or pelvic inflammatory disease. A normal semen analysis obtained after 3 days abstention is sufficient to confirm a normal healthy population of sperm; however, a single suboptimal sample needs repeating to confirm oligospermia and further investigations are necessary until two suboptimal samples have been obtained. If a subsequent sample is normal, then no further action is necessary.

See Chapter 7, *Gynaecology by Ten Teachers*, 18th edition.

17 **True: d.** If the cervical os is open, it is an inevitable miscarriage. If an ultrasound scan shows products of >50 mm. in diameter, one would consider evacuation of retained products of conception. If products are between 30 and 50 mm, one would consider either medical or surgical evacuation of the uterus, and if <30 mm conservative treatment would be appropriate. Serum β-hCG is not useful in dating the pregnancy and levels vary considerably between patients at the same gestation. The snowstorm appearance on ultrasound scan is suggestive of hydatidiform mole pregnancy.

See Chapter 8, *Gynaecology by Ten Teachers*, 18th edition.

18 **True: a, b, c.** Miscarriage is much more likely after the age of 40 (30–40 per cent) compared to under the age of 40 (6–10 per cent). The most common cause of spontaneous miscarriage is a spontaneous chromosomal defect.

See Chapter 8, *Gynaecology by Ten Teachers*, 18th edition.

19 **True: a, b, d.** Ultrasound is very useful in assessing molar pregnancy. There is a typical 'snowstorm' appearance but with partial molar pregnancies, one can also see a fetus. Histology is used to confirm the diagnosis. Partial molar pregnancies are usually triploid, having two sets of chromosomes from the paternal origin and one from maternal origin. Most have a 69XXX or 69XXY gene type.

See Chapter 8, *Gynaecology by Ten Teachers*, 18th edition.

20 **True: c, d.** The incidence of ectopic pregnancy is 22 per 1000 live births and 16 per 1000 pregnancies. Ectopic pregnancy is associated with chlamydial infection and methotrexate is contraindicated if the mass is >2 cm in diameter.

See Chapter 8, *Gynaecology by Ten Teachers*, 18th edition.

21 **True: a, b.** The outpouching of columnar epithelium on to the ectocervix is termed as cervical ectropion or ectopy. An erosion is a common misnomer, which should be avoided, as it conveys the impression of eroded tissue on the surface of the cervix which is incorrect. Columnar epithelium undergoes metaplasia to a normal squamous epithelium. The change of one normal cell type to another cell type is termed metaplasia, whereas dysplasia describes transformation from a normal cell type to an abnormal cell type (e.g. cervical intraepithelium neoplasia).

Vaginal discharge and postcoital bleeding should always be seen as pathological until proven otherwise. Other causes of vaginal discharge need to be excluded prior to treatment with cold coagulation. High vaginal swabs for bacterial vaginosis and endocervical swabs for chlamydia and gonorrhoea need to be taken and colposcopy needs to be undertaken if the patient does not have normal cytology on smear. A physiological vaginal discharge and postcoital bleeding are often seen with an ectopy, but a cervical malignancy or infective lesion need to be excluded prior to treatment with cold coagulation or, occasionally, some clinicians will use a gel to alter the vaginal pH which can shrink an ectropion.

See Chapter 9, *Gynaecology by Ten Teachers*, 18th edition.

22 **True: a, d, e.** Dermoid cysts are lined by either ectodermal tissue, such as skin, sebum or hair, or by endodermal tissue, such as bone or teeth. Typically, only 10 per cent of dermoids are bilateral.

See Chapter 11, *Gynaecology by Ten Teachers*, 18th edition.

23 **True: a, c, d, e.** Call–Exner bodies are pathognomonic of granulosa cell tumours.

See Chapter 11, *Gynaecology by Ten Teachers*, 18th edition.

24 **True: c, d.** Single cysts with no suspicious features tend not to be malignant. Multiple cysts located round the periphery with a dense stroma are pathognomonic of polycystic ovary syndrome. Calcification and fat are often suggestive of a dermoid cyst, which is benign.

See Chapter 11, *Gynaecology by Ten Teachers*, 18th edition.

25 **True: b.** Cervical cancer is the second commonest cancer in women worldwide; breast cancer being the commonest. There are approximately 1500 deaths in England and Wales from carcinoma of the cervix; however, the rate has fallen steeply in recent years owing to the introduction of the cervical cytology screening programme. HPV type 16 and 18 are the most commonly associated with cervical cancer. Cervical cancer is associated with previous HPV infection.

See Chapter 12, *Gynaecology by Ten Teachers*, 18th edition.

26 **True: a, b, e.** Cervical cytology is inaccurate in pregnancy and should be deferred until 12 weeks postpartum. The cervical screening programme only screens for squamous cervical intraepithelial neoplasia. Occasionally, abnormalities of the glandular epithelia are detected (cervical glandular intraepithelial neoplasia; CGIN) but can also be missed if they occur high up the cervical canal.

See Chapter 12, *Gynaecology by Ten Teachers*, 18th edition.

27 **True: b, d.**

See Chapter 12, *Gynaecology by Ten Teachers*, 18th edition.

28 **True: a, b, e.** Nulliparity and late menopause are risk factors for endometrial cancer along with ovarian tumour, previous pelvic irradiation and a family history of breast, ovary or colon cancer.

See Chapter 12, *Gynaecology by Ten Teachers*, 18th edition.

29 **True: b, d.** Preclinical invasive disease of a depth of <3 mm and a width of 7 mm can be treated with a LLETZ. With any greater depth, there is a risk of lymph nodal involvement and local spread; therefore, a radical hysterectomy should be performed. A Wertheim's hysterectomy involves removal of the uterus, cervix, paracervical tissue and lymph nodes, and the upper third of the vagina. Poor bladder emptying may be a consequence of a Wertheim's hysterectomy owing to division of the parasympathetic nerve supply to the bladder, which runs in the uterosacral ligaments.

See Chapter 12, *Gynaecology by Ten Teachers*, 18th edition.

30 **True: d.** Carcinoma of the ovary is common in wealthy countries. It does have a similar incidence to carcinoma of the endometrium but has a much greater mortality. The peak age is 50–60 and is rare at an age of <35. The mainstay of treatment is surgery and chemotherapy with cisplatin and paclitaxol or carboplatin.

See Chapter 13, *Gynaecology by Ten Teachers*, 18th edition.

31 **True: b, c.**

See Chapter 13, *Gynaecology by Ten Teachers*, 18th edition.

32 **True: a, d.** Late menopause is associated with ovarian cancer and the combined pill is protective against ovarian cancer with a lifetime instance of 4 times less than those not using the pill. Implanon has no effect on the development of ovarian carcinoma.

See Chapter 13, *Gynaecology by Ten Teachers*, 18th edition.

33 **True: b, e.** In the normal population, there is a lifetime risk of developing ovarian cancer of 1 per cent. If a patient has one relative with ovarian cancer, their risk remains at 1–2 per cent. If a patient has two first-order affected relatives, their risk increases to 10 per cent.

See Chapter 13, *Gynaecology by Ten Teachers*, 18th edition.

34 **All are true.** Computerized tomography (CT) allows visualization of local invasion and spread to lymph nodes. Barium enema and IVP evaluate tumour invasion into the rectum and descending colon and ureteric obstruction (although these are less commonly required). Ultrasound assesses the nature, size and location of the cyst along with CT. CA 125 is a non-specific tumour marker used to monitor treatment of ovarian cancer.

See Chapter 13, *Gynaecology by Ten Teachers*, 18th edition.

35 **True: a, c, d.** Cisplatin has a number of well-documented side effects, which include renal damage. However, the nephrotoxicity can be prevented by the use of vigorous diuresis. Cumulative dose-related neurotoxicity manifests as paraesthesia and ototoxicity.

See Chapter 13, *Gynaecology by Ten Teachers*, 18th edition.

36 **True: a, d.** Theca cell tumours and androblastomas are both sex-cord stroma tumours. Teratoma is a germ cell tumour.

See Chapter 13, *Gynaecology by Ten Teachers*, 18th edition.

37 **True: c, d.** The peak age of instance is <30 years old. CA 125 is elevated in epithelial cell tumours, not dysgerminomas. Immature teratoma is malignant and the benign form is a mature teratoma, which is called a dermoid.

See Chapter 13, *Gynaecology by Ten Teachers*, 18th edition.

38 **True: a, c, e.** Although some systemic diseases such as diabetes are associated with pruritis vulvae, nephrotic syndrome is not. Vaginal discharge may be concurrent but is not a cause of pruritis vulvae.

See Chapter 14, *Gynaecology by Ten Teachers*, 18th edition.

39 **True: b, c, d.** Lichen sclerosis commonly affects the labia minora and the perianal region. Dark red and brown pigmentation is more suggestive of vulval intraepithelial neoplasia.

See Chapter 14, *Gynaecology by Ten Teachers*, 18th edition.

40 **True: b, c.** Primary syphilis causes vulval ulcers but tertiary syphilis causes neurosyphilis. HPV is not associated with vulval ulcers, but is associated with cervical intraepithelial neoplasia and cervical cancer. Ulcerative colitis does not cause benign vulval ulcers, however, Crohn's disease does.

See Chapter 14, *Gynaecology by Ten Teachers*, 18th edition.

41 **True: c, d.** The lower genital tract is lined by simple cuboidal epithelium in the pre-pubertal state and changes to stratified squamous under the influence of oestrogen. Oestrogen causes the vaginal pH to be reduced to around 3.5–4.5. Bacterial vaginosis is the commonest cause of abnormal vaginal discharge in women of childbearing age.

See Chapter 15, *Gynaecology by Ten Teachers*, 18th edition.

42 **True: b.** Diagnosis of herpes simplex is made after collection of serum from vesicles. This is then analysed by electron microscopy or monolayer tissue culture. Reactivation does arise in the dorsal root ganglia. Secondary infection in pregnancy does not require delivery by lower segment Caesarean section as vertical transmission cannot occur. The fetus develops passive immunity from maternal antibodies that cross the placenta. If there is a primary infection near term, then delivery of the infant would be by Caesarean section. Antiviral treatment is not useful in established disease, as secondary infection usually resolves in the same time as viral treatment would work.

See Chapter 15, *Gynaecology by Ten Teachers*, 18th edition.

43 **True: a, d.** The most sensitive and specific test for syphilis is fluorescent treponemal antibody (FTA). This requires a skilled interpretation and most laboratories perform the *Treponema pallidum* haemagglutination assay (TPHA) or *Treponema pallidum* particle agglutination (TPPA) test instead. A non-specific test, such as the Venereal Disease Research Laboratory test (VDRL), is often used in addition. Usually primary syphilis presents as a painless ulcer (chancre) with occasional regional lymph node enlargement. Treatment for syphilis is with simple penicillin.

See Chapter 15, *Gynaecology by Ten Teachers*, 18th edition.

44 True: b, c. Stress incontinence is a symptom of an involuntary loss of urine when the patient coughs or sneezes. It is not a diagnosis. Urodynamic stress incontinence (USI) is a diagnosis that is gained on filling cystometry, if the patient leaks with a rise in intra-abdominal pressure but with no subsequent rise in detrusor pressure. Detrusor overactivity is idiopathic in 85 per cent of cases; however, it may be caused by neuropathy, incontinence surgery or outflow obstruction. Stress urinary incontinence results from poor suburethral support and descent at the bladder neck and proximal urethra.

A total of 10–15 per cent of women have a poor urinary stream. This can be either due to urethral obstruction, which can be as a result of scarring from previous surgery, or extraurethral compression (e.g. gravid uterus, ovarian cyst or fibroid). However, poor voiding may also be secondary to a weak detrusor muscle. The only way to distinguish between the two is to perform pressure flow studies on the patient. Urethral obstruction will have a high pressure–low flow picture, whereas a poor detrusor muscle will have a low pressure–low flow picture.

See Chapter 16, *Gynaecology by Ten Teachers*, 18th edition.

45 True: c, e. Pelvic organ prolapse is predominantly found in multiparous women. The risk of prolapse increases with increasing parity. Pelvic organ prolapse affects around 2 per cent of nulliparous women and this suggests a congenital predisposition in these women despite them not undergoing childbirth. Epidural alone is not a risk factor for the development of prolapse; however, forceps macrosomia and malposition of the baby are all associated with traumatic delivery and subsequent development of prolapse.

See Chapter 17, *Gynaecology by Ten Teachers*, 18th edition.

46 True: c, d. The follicles are located peripherally around the cortex of the ovary with the central medulla being heavily vascularized. The central medulla is mesenchymal in origin. In a woman's lifetime she will only have around 400 follicles that will ovulate.

See Chapter 18, *Gynaecology by Ten Teachers*, 18th edition.

47 True: a, d. Androgens are converted to oestrogen by an enzyme called aromatase. The process is known as aromatization. Granulosa cells are stimulated by FSH in the developing follicle and, once ovulation has occurred, thecal cells produce oestrogen from androgens under the stimulating effect of LH. Initially, the levels of inhibin produced by the ovary start to fall around the menopause. This glycoprotein inhibits FSH production by the pituitary gland and, therefore, plasma FSH starts to rise around the menopause. It is only in the true postmenopausal state can one measure consistently elevated FSH levels, which helps with the diagnosis of the menopause.

See Chapter 18, *Gynaecology by Ten Teachers*, 18th edition.

48 True: b, d. Provided there is a normal-sized uterus, vaginal hysterectomy can often be performed and extensive prolapse is not necessary. Vaginal hysterectomy is associated with a quicker recovery. This is due to the absence of an abdominal incision which causes much greater pain than a vaginal incision. Vaginal hysterectomy is associated with a high risk of haematoma formation. The risk of ureteric injury is higher with abdominal surgery.

49 True: c, d. The gestation should not exceed 24 weeks. The request for termination can only be carried out after two registered medical practitioners independently consider the effects of continuation of the pregnancy and feel that the woman has formed a judgement that termination is in her best interest. It is recommended that termination should be performed after 8 weeks' gestation, as the chance of missing fetal products and the pregnancy continuing are higher if the pregnancy is less than 8 weeks.

Chapter 7

Short answer questions

Normal and abnormal sexual development and puberty

1 **A 17-year-old girl presents complaining she hasn't started having periods yet. What are the salient features in the history and examination that would help to determine a diagnosis?**

History

Developmental history: reflects sexual hormone production.
Presence/absence of cyclical symptoms: suggests ovarian function normal.
History of chronic illness: inhibits hypothalamic–pituitary–ovarian axis
Excessive weight loss/eating disorder: inhibits hypothalamic–pituitary–ovarian axis.
Excessive exercise: inhibits hypothalamic–pituitary–ovarian axis.
Contraceptive history: menses on exogenous hormones may mask primary amenorrhoea.
Reproductive history: pregnancy is the commonest cause of secondary amenorrhoea.

Menopausal symptoms and family history of premature menopause: may be familial.
Medications: can inhibit hypothalamic–pituitary–ovarian axis, e.g. gonadotrophin-releasing hormone (GnRH) analogues.
Virilizing signs, galactorrhoea: suggests androgen tumour, congenital adrenal hyperplasia (CAH), prolactinoma.
Hirsutism, acne: may be suggestive of polycystic ovarian syndrome (PCOS).   (12 marks)

Examination

Height: short stature associated with chromosomal abnormality, e.g. Turner's syndrome.
Weight/body mass index (BMI): polycystic ovary syndrome associated with raised BMI.

Secondary sexual characteristics/evidence of virilization:
Visual fields: ~~homonymous~~ bitemporal hemianopia associated with pituitary tumour.
Pelvic examination: imperforate hymen, absent pelvic organs.   (5 marks)

See Chapter 3, *Gynaecology by Ten Teachers*, 18th edition.

2 **Write short notes on the five stages of puberty.**

The events that occur in changes from a child to adult female usually occur in the following sequence:

1 Growth spurt
2 Breast development
3 Pubic hair growth
4 Menstruation
5 Axillary hair growth

The above sequence of events occurs in around 70 per cent of girls but there may be minor differences in timing. Tanner has described pubertal development in five stages. (3 marks)

The growth spurt starts at around 11 years of age owing to the effect of oestrogen and most girls have reached their final height by the age of 15 with the fusion of the femoral endplate. (2 marks)

Breast bud development starts after the growth spurt in response to the production of oestradiol by the ovary. This is due to an increase in the production of GnRH from the pituitary gland. In initial breast development, the areola tissue appears more pronounced and then the breast tissue grows to become more confluent with the areola as it develops. (2 marks)

Menarche is defined as the first menstrual period and occurs at any age between 9 and 17 years. Initially periods can be very irregular and it can take from 5 to 8 years from the time of menarche for women to develop a regular cycle after full maturation of the hypothalamic–pituitary–ovarian axis. (3 marks)

Pubic hair growth initially begins on the labia and then gradually extends over the mons pubis. Axillary hair growth is a late development. (2 marks)

See Chapter 3, *Gynaecology by Ten Teachers*, 18th edition.

Disorders of the menstrual cycle

3 **A 45-year-old woman is referred by her general practitioner (GP) complaining of 'heavy periods'. What are the salient features in her history and examination?**

History
Last menstrual period (LMP)/cycle length
Duration of bleeding
Passage of clots/flooding/number of sanitary protection used and how soaked
Intermenstrual bleeding and postcoital bleeding
Past gynecological history: pelvic inflammatory disease (PID; associated with increased loss), smear history, contraception – intrauterine contraceptive device (IUCD), which increases loss, or contraceptive pill, which regulates and usually decreases loss.
Symptoms of anaemia: lethargy, shortness of breath on exertion, syncope. (4 marks)

Clinical examination

General:
- Endocrine disorders (hirsutism, striae, goitre, skin pigmentation, tremor)
- Secondary sexual characteristics
- Signs of anaemia (tachycardia, pale sclerae)
- Liver disease, clotting disorder (bruising, petichaie)

Abdominal:
- Liver enlargement
- Pelvic mass (?fibroids)

Vagina:
- Signs of trauma, infection
- Visualize cervix for ectopic, malignancy   (4 marks)

3a What investigations would you do if the patient had a regular 28-day cycle and no pelvic mass, and why?
Full blood count (FBC): anaemia, platelet function   (1 mark)

3b What further tests would you do if she had an irregular cycle and why?
Thyroid function tests (TFTs): endocrine *only* if suspicion of thyroid disease
Serum β-human chorionic gonadotrophin (sβ-hCG): only if pregnancy suspected
Serum androgens: only if signs of hirsutism and acne
Prolactin: only if oligomenorrhoea or lactation
Coagulation screen: only if bruising, etc.
Urea and electrolytes (U&Es), liver function tests (LFTs): only if signs of renal/liver impairment

                                                                             (6 marks)

3c What further tests could be done if all the above are normal or not clinically indicated (which is usually the case), and why?
Pelvic ultrasound scan: to assess for fibroids if uterus enlarged or endometrial polyps, if intermenstrual bleeding
Hysteroscopy/endometrial biopsy: as the patient is over the age of 40, Royal College of Obstetricians and Gynaecologists (RCOG) guidelines recommend hysteroscopy and endometrial biopsy to exclude malignancy and assess correlation of endometrial phase with cycle   (2 marks)

See Chapter 5, *Gynaecology by Ten Teachers*, 18th edition.

Fertility control

4 A 25-year-old woman attends the local family planning clinic to discuss various forms of contraception. She has an irregular cycle, has had two partners in the past, but is in a new stable relationship and has one daughter aged 3. What are the salient features within the history and examination that would help you to help her choose one form of contraception over another?
Menstrual cycle: This woman has an irregular cycle but it is important to determine exactly the nature of her bleeding, duration of bleeding and length between periods. It is also important to know whether she has any breakthrough bleeding/intermenstrual bleeding. This can be a sign of infection and chlamydia swabs should be taken.   (3 marks)

Parity/plans for future pregnancies: It is important to know whether this woman plans any further pregnancies or whether her family is complete. Usually it is not recommended for irreversible forms of contraception at this stage as she has just started a new relationship and the incidence of regret following permanent sterilization is much greater in the under 30 age group.   (2 marks)

Sexual history: It is important to know the number of partners this woman has had, whether she has had any previous pelvic infections and whether she is now in a stable relationship. One should ask what forms of contraception she has tried in the past, as some of these may not have agreed with the individual and so would be contraindicated to use again. (2 marks)

General gynaecological history: One should ask about smear history as well as any previous cervical or pelvic surgery.

Drug history: One should check whether the patient is taking any liver enzyme-inducing agents or antibiotics. (2 marks)

Contraindications: Certain forms of contraception would be contraindicated, especially the combined pill. The absolute contraindications to taking the combined oral contraceptive pill are:
- Circulatory disease, ischaemic heart disease, cerebrovascular accidents, significant hypertension, arterial or venous thrombosis, any acquired or inherited thrombotic tendency or any significant risk factors for cardiovascular disease.
- Acute or severe liver disease.
- Oestrogen-dependent neoplasms, particularly breast cancer.
- Focal migraine. (4 marks)

The relative contraindications include:
- Generalized migraine.
- Long-term immobilization.
- Irregular vaginal bleeding, which has not had a diagnosis obtained.
- Less severe risk factors for cardiovascular disease, such as obesity, heavy smoking and diabetes. (4 marks)

Examination: One would want to know the patient's weight, blood pressure as well as a general pelvic examination to assess uterine size and assess for pelvic masses. (1 mark)

See Chapter 6, *Gynaecology by Ten Teachers*, 18th edition.

---

5 **Outline the principal features that one would include in a consent form to women who are considering sterilization in an outpatient appointment.**

Female sterilization is generally performed by occlusion of the Fallopian tubes. This is done either using Filshie clips, plastic rings or with the use of excision and ligation of the tubes. The procedure is performed usually through laparoscopic surgery but can be performed as an open procedure, especially if concurrent surgery is occurring, e.g. Caesarean section. (2 marks)

It is advisable to warn the patient that the procedure should be considered permanent and irreversible. Reversal can be performed, but this is not provided under the National Health Service (NHS) and no guarantees can be given about the success of reversal of sterilization. (2 marks)

Failure of sterilization should be explained and the rate of 1 in 200 should be quoted. Failure rates rise either due to incomplete occlusion of the tubal lumen or recanalization of a previously appropriately occluded lumen. If sterilization fails owing to application of clips in the wrong structure, such as the round ligament, this is indefensible in court. It is, therefore, advisable to take photographs of the tubes once they are occluded at the time of surgery. (3 marks)

The patient should be warned about the increased risk of ectopic pregnancy should they fall pregnant, although this is still very unlikely. (1 mark)

If patients are using the combined oral contraceptive pill, their periods may be artificially light. Once they are sterilized, they will stop taking the combined pill and their periods will return to their physiological status. If the patient has had a history of menorrhagia, then one should warn them that the chance of this recurring is high and alternative contraception, such as the Mirena, may be more appropriate. (1 mark)

All other forms of contraception should be discussed with the patient, including male sterilization, which is safer, does not require a general anaesthetic and has a lower failure rate. (1 mark)

See Chapter 6, *Gynaecology by Ten Teachers*, 18th edition.

Infertility

6 **A couple attend the infertility clinic for the first time having been trying to conceive a pregnancy for the last 12 months of unprotected intercourse. What are the salient points in the history?**

Maternal age: Rates of conception rapidly decline after the age of 35. (1 mark)

Parity and gravidity: ages and modes of delivery of previous pregnancies. (2 marks)

Menstrual cycle: regularity of menstrual cycle suggests but does not confirm ovulation; oligomenorrhoea or amenorrhoea may be suggestive of an ovulatory disorder. (1 mark)

Contraception: previous contraception is important, as some contraceptives, such as the Depo, can have a prolonged effect. (1 mark)

Disorders suggestive of a general endocrine problem: one should list in the history symptoms that may suggest an endocrine disorder that can affect ovulation. (1 mark)

Tubal disease: one should look in the history for risk factors for tubal disease, such as a history of sexually transmitted diseases/PID, pelvic abscesses, previous pelvic or abdominal surgery, tubal surgery, and previous ectopic pregnancies. (2 marks)

General history: one should ask about smear history, rubella status and blood group, if known, as well as discussing pre-conceptual folic acid, which should be taken for 3 months periconception. On general examination, one should look for signs of raised BMI, signs of hirsutism and other endocrine disorders and secondary sexual characteristics. On abdominal examination, one should inspect for signs of previous abdominal/pelvic surgery and vaginal examination should be performed. Swabs should be taken for chlamydia, gonorrhoea and other sexually transmitted diseases, and a smear should be obtained if patient has not had one as part of the normal recall process. (4 marks)

History and examination of male partner: this is essential. One should note age, history of any children in this relationship or other relationships, smoking, alcohol use and occupation. It is important to enquire about testicular trauma, undescended testes, mumps and previous sexually transmitted diseases. On examination, one should assess the size of each testis, check for varicoceles and descent, and note secondary sexual characteristics. One should also discuss quite openly the couple's frequency and timing of coitus to ensure this is occurring during the fertile time of the woman's cycle (i.e. 14 days prior to menstrual period). (4 marks)

See Chapter 7, *Gynaecology by Ten Teachers*, 18th edition.

Disorders of early pregnancy

7 **Write short notes on threatened miscarriage, missed miscarriage and incomplete miscarriage.**

Threatened miscarriage

This is defined as bleeding in early pregnancy of >24 weeks' gestation. The patient presents with vaginal bleeding that may be associated with suprapubic pain. On vaginal examination, the cervical os is closed. Ultrasound demonstrates a gestational sac with a fetal pole and the fetal heart is seen. There may or may not be an intra-uterine haematoma present. (3 marks)

Missed miscarriage

Patients may present either with minimal bleeding, old blood loss or no bleeding at all. Sometimes the diagnosis is made incidentally at ultrasound scan when patients come for a routine 12 week or 20 week scan. The diagnosis is confirmed if ultrasound shows an embryo of <20 weeks with no fetal heart and no signs of expulsion. Alternatively, a gestation sac of >20 mm and no embryo, or a fetal pole of >6 mm with no fetal heart seen would be classified as a missed miscarriage. Management can be either medically induced miscarriage or surgical evacuation. (3 marks)

Incomplete miscarriage

Patients usually present with heavy bleeding and cramping pain, and have partial expulsion of the products of conception. On speculum examination, if the cervical os is open, it is termed an 'inevitable miscarriage'. A transvaginal scan will show products of conception within the uterine cavity. The management can be either expectant, surgical evacuation or medical, and depends on the size of the products of conception within the uterine cavity. As a general rule, if the products of conception are > 50 mm, then surgical or medical evacuation would be recommended. (4 marks)

See Chapter 8, *Gynaecology by Ten Teachers*, 18th edition.

8 **A 20-year-old woman has had an episode of amenorrhoea lasting for 6 weeks and 5 days, having had a previous regular 28-day cycle. She presents with right iliac fossa pain and light vaginal bleeding. She has had a previous history of chlamydia but no other medical illnesses, and is not taking any medication. On examination, she is in pain and distressed. The patient's pulse is 89 beats per minute, she had a blood pressure of 120/70 mmHg. Abdominal examination and vaginal examination exhibited tenderness in the right iliac fossa with guarding. She was also tender in the right adnexum on vaginal examination. Urinary pregnancy test was positive. What are the possible differential diagnoses and what investigations would you perform and why?**

Ectopic pregnancy is the most likely diagnosis that needs to be excluded before any other diagnosis can be made. Other possible diagnoses that need to be considered include appendicitis, corpus luteum/ovarian cyst pain and threatened miscarriage. (4 marks)

A full blood count should be obtained to assess if the patient is anaemic. If there has been any concealed bleeding into the peritoneal cavity of any significance, a full blood count will show a drop in the haemoglobin. A tachycardia may be attributed to anaemia but also may be due to her pain and distress. (2 marks)

Blood should be taken to determine blood group, and serum saved and cross-matched in case the patient requires subsequent surgery or transfusion. If the patient is rhesus negative and has a surgical intervention, she may require anti-D prophylaxis. (1 mark)

The maternal sβhCG levels should be quantified and can be useful in raising suspicions for an ectopic pregnancy, if ultrasound scan shows an empty uterus and the sβhCG is >1000 IU/L. (1 mark)

An ultrasound scan should be arranged to assess whether there is a viable intrauterine pregnancy. The adnexae can also be assessed for masses/ovarian cysts as well as looking for other suspicious features, such as free fluid in the pouch of Douglas, which would correlate with internal bleeding. (2 marks)

The most likely diagnosis is an ectopic pregnancy. In view of the patient's distress, she requires an urgent diagnostic laparoscopy. If this demonstrated an ectopic pregnancy, then the surgeon should proceed to a salpingectomy if the contralateral tube looks normal or salpingostomy if the contralateral Fallopian tube looks diseased.

(2 marks)

See Chapter 8, *Gynaecology by Ten Teachers*, 18th edition.

Benign diseases of the uterus and cervix

9 Write short notes on the principles of a screening programme.

There are ten principles of screening that are now adopted by the World Health Organisation.

1 The condition should be an important health problem. (1 mark)
2 There should be a recognizable latent or early symptomatic stage. (1 mark)
3 The natural history of the condition, including development from latent to declared disease, should be adequately understood. (1 mark)
4 There should be an accepted treatment for patients with recognized disease and early intervention will alter prognosis compared with treatment of later manifested disease. (1 mark)
5 There should be a suitable test or examination. (1 mark)
6 The test should be acceptable to the population. (1 mark)
7 There should be an agreed policy on whom to treat as patients. (1 mark)
8 Facilities for diagnosis and treatment should be available. (1 mark)
9 The cost of screening (including diagnosis and treatment of patients diagnosed) should be economically balanced in relation to possible expenditure to medical care of patients with declared disease. (1 mark)
10 Screening should be a continuing process and not a 'once and for all' project. (1 mark)

See Chapter 9, *Gynaecology by Ten Teachers*, 18th edition.

Endometriosis and adenomyosis

10 Outline the four theories for the pathophysiology of endometriosis.

1 *Menstrual regurgitation and implantation.* One theory is that endometriosis occurs as a result of retrograde menstruation and that implantation of endometrial glands and tissue occurs into the peritoneal surface. This has been shown to occur in experimental models. (2 marks)
2 *Coelomic epithelium transformation.* Another theory is that peritoneal cells and cells in the ovary which are derived from the Mullerian duct undergo dedifferentiation back to their primitive origin and then transform into endometrial cells. It is not yet known what might stimulate this dedifferentiation. (2 marks)
3 *Genetic and immunological factors.* Some women of certain genetic/immunological predisposition may possess factors that render them susceptible to the development of endometriosis. This is substantiated by a familial tendency as well as racial tendencies. (2 marks)
4 *Vascular lymphatic spread.* Occasionally endometriosis can be found inside and outside the peritoneal cavity, such as skin, kidney and lung. This may occur due to embolization of endometrial tissue via vascular lymphatic channels or at surgery. (2 marks)

See Chapter 10, *Gynaecology by Ten Teachers*, 18th edition.

11 A GP refers a 30-year-old woman with menorrhagia and pelvic pain. He suggests she may have endometriosis. What are the salient features in her history and on clinical examination? What are the possible differential diagnoses? What investigations would you perform to confirm the diagnosis?

History

The salient features include dysmenorrhoea, the demonstration of cyclical pelvic pain, deep dyspareunia, a history of subfertility or infertility. Bladder symptoms may include cyclical haematuria or ureteric obstruction, and bowel symptoms may include cyclical rectal bleeding or pain on defaecation. (3 marks)

Examination

One would try and elicit pain in the pouch of Douglas by palpation over the rectovaginal septum and uterosacral ligaments. It is sometimes possible to palpate nodules of endometriosis on rectovaginal examination. Bidigital examination may help palpate any pelvic masses such as endometriomas. (3 marks)

Differential diagnoses

These would be adenomyosis, pelvic inflammatory disease or bowel pathology (irritable bowel syndrome). (1 mark)

Investigations

These would include an ultrasound scan to exclude any endometriomata. A CA 125 is of little clinical use but may be slightly raised in endometriosis. A diagnostic laparoscopy with or without tubal patency testing will confirm a diagnosis of endometriosis, and endometrial explants can be seen within the peritoneal cavity. (4 marks)

See Chapter 10, *Gynaecology by Ten Teachers*, 18th edition.

12 Write short notes on the differences in epidemiology, symptomatology, investigation and treatment of endometriosis and adenomyosis.

Adenomyosis tends to affect women between the age of 30 and 40, whereas endometriosis tends to affect women in their late 20s and 30s. (2 marks)

Women with adenomyosis present with increasingly severe secondary spasmodic dysmenorrhoea and increased menorrhagia. On examination, they tend to have a tender uterus, particularly pre-menstrually. In women with an endometrioma, tenderness is usually elicited in the pouch of Douglas, rectovaginal septum and adnexae. (3 marks)

The diagnosis of adenomyosis can sometimes be suspected on ultrasound, if there is asymmetrical irregular echogenicity within the myometrium. Magnetic resonance imaging provides further enhanced images and is the investigation of choice. If the patient has endometriosis, ultrasound may demonstrate the presence of endometriomas. The diagnosis of adenomyosis can only truly be made at hysterectomy, as it is a histological finding. (3 marks)

Endometriosis can be treated by simple analgesia. Inhibition of ovulation using the combined oral contraceptive pill and GnRH analogues can give symptomatic relief. Ablation, resection or total abdominal hysterectomy and bilateral salpingo-oophorectomy are more definitive. Adenomyosis is treated definitively by hysterectomy. (2 marks)

See Chapter 10, *Gynaecology by Ten Teachers*, 18th edition.

Benign diseases of the ovary

13 Outline the different strategies for the management of a single 4 cm ovarian cyst in the pre-menopausal, pregnant and postmenopausal woman.

Pre-menopausal

Cysts on the ovary can be physiological, benign or malignant. Physiological cysts usually measure less than 40 cm. Physiological cysts are more common in this age group. An ultrasound and CA 125 may help differentiate whether the cyst is sinister or pathological. Sinister findings would be septae, solid elements or large cysts. If the cyst appears suspicious and may or may not have elevated tumour markers, discussion at a multidisciplinary meeting is advisable to decide on whether surgery is indicated and what procedure would be most appropriate. If the cyst is symptomatic (painful), then treatment either by laparoscopy or laparotomy would be warranted.

(4 marks)

Pregnant

Cysts are often found asymptomatically at ultrasound, at antenatal clinic or at Caesarean section. The risk of torsion is increased in pregnancy due to the movement of the pelvic organs out of the pelvis as the gravid uterus grows. Ultrasound monitoring during each trimester is sufficient provided the patient remains asymptomatic. Surgery should be avoided until 14 weeks to reduce the risk of miscarriage and intervention with a corpus luteum, which should have regressed by 12 weeks. Surgery is usually contemplated if the patient's symptoms are serious, such as significant pain, cyst rupture and significant bleeding or torsion. Tocolysis is often used at the time of surgery to reduce the risk of miscarriage and pre-term labour.

(4 marks)

Postmenopausal

Physiological cysts on the ovary are unlikely in the postmenopause but can still be found. Evaluation of the cyst using ultrasound, CA 125, Doppler and the patient's age can be entered into an equation to give a risk of malignancy (relative malignancy index; RMI). If the risk of malignancy score is low and the patient is asymptomatic, they can be left alone with no further follow-up. If the malignancy score is high, then referral and discussion through a multidisciplinary team meeting should be arranged, with possible subsequent hysterectomy and bilateral oopherectomy, if malignancy is suspected.

(4 marks)

See Chapter 11, *Gynaecology by Ten Teachers*, 18th edition.

Benign diseases of the ovary

14 **A 40-year-old patient presents with a history of ovarian cysts in the past. She is admitted with acute abdominal pain after 2 weeks of pelvic discomfort and urinary frequency. On examination, there is a mass palpable arising out of the pelvis. What is the differential diagnosis? What are the salient features in the history and examination, and how would you investigate the patient?**

The most likely differential diagnoses would include a benign ovarian cyst, cyst rupture or torsion, urinary retention, fibroids (possibly degenerating). Other less likely diagnoses would include appendicitis with appendix abscess, PID/pyo-/hydrosalpinx. (3 marks)

Salient features in the history would include the last menstrual period (if late exclude pregnancy) and cycle length, contraception, previous ovarian cysts or fibroids, sexual history, pain (whether this was associated with vomiting or rigors as this may be suggestive of appendicitis/torsion/PID). Shoulder-tip pain or bleeding may be indicative of ectopic pregnancy.

(3 marks)

On ultrasound, benign cysts tend to be large and unilocular simple cysts, whereas malignant tumours have septae, often solid or semisolid, and are larger. A raised CA 125 is strongly suggestive of ovarian carcinoma, but can also be mildly elevated in endometriosis and pelvic inflammatory disease. If ultrasound and CA 125 suggest a malignancy, a computerized tomography scan is mandatory to evaluate further the nature of the cyst as well as nodal spread. (4 marks)

See Chapter 11, *Gynaecology by Ten Teachers*, 18th edition.

Malignant disease of the uterus and cervix

15 **A 65-year-old woman presents in clinic with a single episode of postmenopausal bleeding. Write short notes on the investigation and management of such a patient.**

The likely differential diagnoses include atrophic vaginal tissues, endometrial polyp or endometrial carcinoma. (3 marks)

Initial investigations involve examination of the lower genital tract looking for atrophic tissues, as well as bimanual examination to assess uterine size and feel for parametrial thickening, which would be suggestive of malignancy. (3 marks)

Pelvic ultrasound scan is useful to measure endometrial thickness and, if this is <4 mm, the patient can be reassured that the risk of malignancy is almost zero, providing they have only had a single episode of postmenopausal bleeding. In this instance, the patients can be discharged but should reattend if they have any further bleeding. Outpatient hysteroscopy and Pipelle aspiration of the endometrium is useful if the endometrial thickness is >4 mm. Rigid saline hysteroscopy occasionally needs to be performed under general anaesthesia for patients who cannot tolerate outpatient hysteroscopy. Another indication for rigid saline hysteroscopy would be if the patient has findings on ultrasound suggestive of a polyp, which cannot be removed in the outpatient setting. (4 marks)

Treatment would depend on the cause. If the patient has atrophic tissues, then topical oestrogens are appropriate. A polypectomy can be utilized, if there is a single polyp that is benign, and the mainstay of treatment for endometrial carcinoma is total abdominal hysterectomy and bilateral salpingo-oophorectomy with or without postoperative radiotherapy. Bilateral pelvic lymph nodes and para-aortic node sampling is often performed, if there are concerns regarding malignancy. (3 marks)

See Chapter 12, *Gynaecology by Ten Teachers*, 18th edition.

Carcinoma of the ovary and Fallopian tube

16 Write short notes on the classification of epithelioid tumours of the ovary.

Epithelioid tumours can be classified into serous, mucinous, endometrioid, clear cell, Brenner and undifferentiated tumours. (1 mark)

With regard to serous tumours, the majority have solid and cystic elements, are often bilateral and have psam-
moma bodies present on histology. (2 marks)

Mucinous tumours account for 10 per cent of the malignant tumours of the ovary. They are usually multilocu-
lar thin-walled cysts with a smooth surface full of mucinous fluid. Mucinous cysts often have exceedingly large
dimensions. (2 marks)

Endometrioid tumours resemble the endometrium of the uterus in histology. They are often cystic unilocular
cysts containing turbid, brown fluid. A total of 15 per cent are associated with an endometrial cancer of the
uterus. (2 marks)

Clear cell tumours are the least common epithelial tumours and often coexist with endometrioid tumours or
endometriosis. (2 marks)

Borderline tumours account for 10 per cent of ovarian tumours. They are usually confined to the ovary and have
a better prognosis. (1 mark)

See Chapter 13, *Gynaecology by Ten Teachers*, 18th edition.

Infections in gynaecology

17 Write short notes on candida, bacterial vaginosis and trichomoniasis vaginalis.

Candida
This is a fungal infection usually caused by the *Candida albicans* organism in 80 per cent of women. It is not sexu-
ally transmitted and women usually present with an itchy sore vagina and vulva, and a curdy white discharge.
Topical treatment is usually sufficient with clotrimazole 500 mg, although oral fluconazole is an alternative.

(3 marks)

Bacterial vaginosis
This is not a sexually transmitted disease. It is typically caused by anaerobic organisms, such as *Gardnerella vagi-
nalis*, *Bacteroides*, *Mobiluncus* and *Micoplasma*. Women typically present with an offensive fishy discharge.
Diagnosis is made on composite Ansel criteria. These criteria are: (1) a pH of 4.5; (2) a fishy smell on the application of potassium hydrochloride; (3) 'clue' cells on microscopy and it is treated with either oral or topical
metronidazole. There is an increased risk of second trimester miscarriage and preterm labour, and women with
a history of this should be screened and treated for the organisms. (4 marks)

Trichomoniasis vaginalis
This is a sexually transmitted disease, the incidence of which is falling in the UK. Women usually present with a
yellow or green discharge. Examination of the cervix shows multiple punctate haemorrhages, which gives the
characteristic 'strawberry' cervix. The diagnosis is made after culturing organisms in Fireberg Whittington
medium. The treatment of choice is metronidazole. (3 marks)

See Chapter 15, *Gynaecology by Ten Teachers*, 18th edition.

Urogynaecology

18 A 35-year-old woman presents with a 2-year history of involuntary loss of urine on exercise and cough-ing. Write short notes on the salient features in her history and examination. What investigations would you arrange and why?

History

Urinary symptoms suggestive of stress incontinence: When and how much does the patient leak? How many pads does the patient use (how many during the day, how many during the night)? (2 marks)

Urinary symptoms suggestive of detrusor overactivity: Does the patient leak at night? Does the patient complain of urgency, urge incontinence, frequency and nocturia? (2 marks)

Voiding symptoms: Are there any voiding difficulties, such as poor urinary stream, incomplete micturition or deviated stream? (1 mark)

Bowel symptoms: constipation, perineal splinting, digitations, irritable bowel. (1 mark)

Past gynaecological history: any relevant previous surgery (e.g. colposuspension). (1 mark)

Past obstetric history: particular relevance should be noted to previous deliveries, the mode of delivery and the birth weight of each child, as stress incontinence is associated with trauma to the pelvic floor (macrosomia, forceps) (1 mark)

Examination

General examination: patient's BMI, nicotine-stained fingers (suggestive of smoking), and abdominal palpation for abdominal and pelvic masses.
Vaginal examination: Particular attention should be paid to look for atrophic changes in the lower genital tract and prolapse. Stress incontinence should also be demonstrated by asking the patient to cough. (2 marks)

Investigations

Mid-stream urine: to exclude urinary tract infection.
Urinary diary: to record the patient's fluid intake and output. This can help to note the patient's functional capacity and the severity of incontinence episodes, as well as educating the patient about their bladder habits.
Pad test: This can help quantify urine loss.
Uroflowmetry and video-cystourethography: Uroflowmetry is performed as part of urodynamic assessment and will help assess the patient's voiding and exclude a voiding difficulty. Cystometry can be performed either by using saline or a radio-opaque filling medium, and video-cystourethography can then be performed. This will diagnose urodynamic stress incontinence, if leakage occurs as a result of coughing in the absence of a rise in detrusor pressure, and detrusor overactivity, if the detrusor pressure rises inappropriately associated with urgency symptoms. (4 marks)

See Chapter 16, *Gynaecology by Ten Teachers,* 18th edition.

The menopause

19 Outline the effects of the menopause and its hypo-oestrogenic state on a woman's physiology.

Symptoms of the menopause are usually stimulated by a fall in circulating oestrogen and may occur prior to the absolute level defined at the postmenopause of <100pmol/L. Symptoms include tiredness, hot flushes, night sweats, insomnia, vaginal dryness and urinary frequency. (3 marks)

Various physiological changes occur and these can affect different systems of the body. The predominant systems affected are the skeletal and cardiovascular systems. Oestrogen acts to prevent bone turnover by balancing the equilibrium between bone resorption and bone formation. A low circulating oestrogen is associated with a greater bone resorption rate over bone formation in the trabecular bone. Trabecular bone has a higher surface area, thus postmenopausal women are at particular risk of osteopaenia and osteoporosis. They are also at higher risk of traumatic fractures, typically of the distal radius and neck of femur.

(3 marks)

The cardiovascular system is the second major physiological system affected in the postmenopausal period and the incidence of myocardial infarction rises significantly at this time. A hypo-oestrogenic state is associated by significant changes in the lipid profile that predisposes women to atheroma. These include raised total cholesterol, lower HDL (high-density lipoprotein) cholesterol and a high LDL (low-density lipoprotein). Triglycerides remain at similar levels to those in the pre-menopausal state. Oestrogen also causes vasoconstriction, owing to reduction in the production of nitrogen synthase. Large randomized controlled trials have shown no benefit and possibly a deleterious effect on the cardiovascular system with the administration of hormone replacement therapy; therefore it is not recommended to start this as a treatment or prevention of cardiovascular disease.

(4marks)

See Chapter 18, *Gynaecology by Ten Teachers*, 18th edition.

Objective structured clinical examination questions

1 History and examination

Outline a format for a gynaecological history, including headings and subheadings.

2 History and examination

Name the two devices seen in Figures 8.1 and 8.2, and outline the patient's position for examination with each, along with their clinical applications.

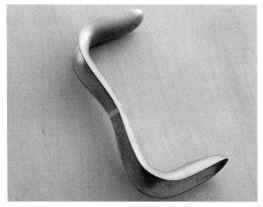

Figure 8.1 Reproduced from Monga A (ed) *Gynaecology By Ten Teachers*, 18th edition. London: Edward Arnold 2006.

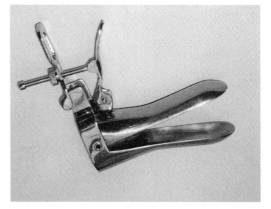

Figure 8.2 Reproduced from Monga A (ed) *Gynaecology By Ten Teachers*, 18th edition. London: Edward Arnold 2006.

3 Embryology, anatomy and physiology

Label the diagrams below of the human female pelvis (Figures 8.3 and 8.4).

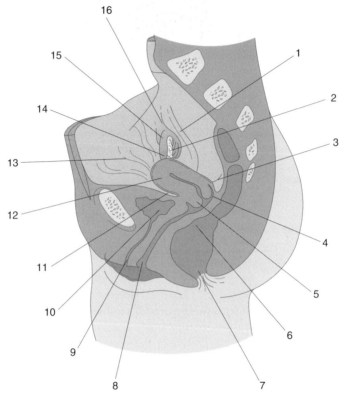

Figure 8.3 Adapted from Monga A (ed) *Gynaecology By Ten Teachers*, 18th edition. London: Edward Arnold 2006.

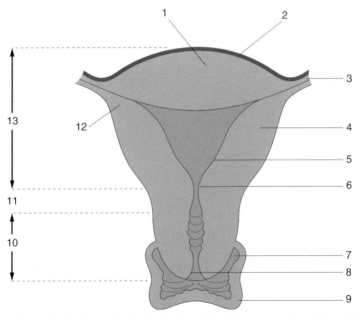

Figure 8.4 Adapted from Monga A (ed) *Gynaecology By Ten Teachers*, 18th edition. London: Edward Arnold 2006.

4 Normal and abnormal sexual development and puberty

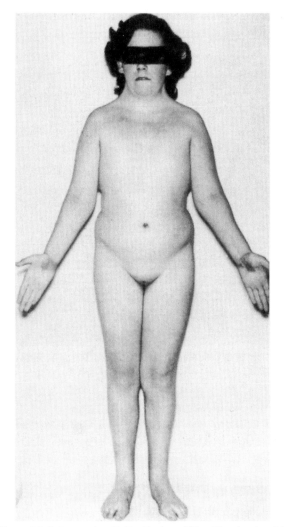

Figure 8.5 Reproduced from Monga A (ed) *Gynaecology By Ten Teachers*, 18th edition. London: Edward Arnold 2006.

a) What clinical condition is demonstrated in this photograph?
b) What is the typical karyotype?
c) What are the typical clinical features?
d) What is the typical hormone profile of this patient?
e) What is the macroscopic appearance of the ovaries at laparotomy for this condition?
f) What are the two phases of treatment for this patient?

5 The normal menstrual cycle

Draw the menstrual cycle outlining changes in the hypothalamic, pituitary and ovarian hormone levels as well as the effect on the endometrium.

6 The normal menstrual cycle

Label these histology sections of endometrium (Figure 8.6a and b) and match the characteristics with each phase.

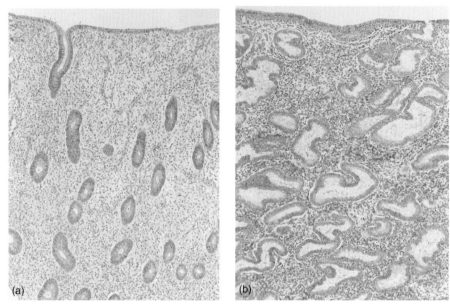

Figure 8.6   Illustrations kindly provided by Dr Colin Stewart; reproduced from Monga A (ed) *Gynaecology By Ten Teachers*, 18th edition. London: Edward Arnold 2006.

Phase:
- Follicular phase
- Secretory phase
- Luteal phase
- Proliferative phase

Characteristics:
- Stromal oedema and glandular growth
- Glandular and stromal proliferation
- Pre-ovulation
- Postovulation
- Progesterone predominates
- Oestrogen predominates

7 Fertility control

List the various methods of contraception along with their failure rate per 100 per women years.

8 Fertility control

A 16-year-old girl attends a clinic having forgotten to take her pill 14 hours ago. How would you counsel her?

9 Fertility control

List the mode of action of the following contraceptives:
- Combined oral contraceptive pill
- Progesterone-only pill
- Depo
- Intrauterine device (IUD)
- Intrauterine system (IUS)
- Condoms
- Natural family planning
- Female sterilization
- Male sterilization

10 Infertility

A couple are referred to the infertility clinic having been trying to conceive a pregnancy after 2 years of unprotected intercourse. Mrs Smith is 29, has irregular periods (2–3 per year), she weighs 16 stone, has significant acne and facial hair. She has no history of pelvic surgery or pelvic infections. Mr Smith has a normal semen analysis and has children from a previous relationship. The investigations from the female partner are as follows:

Day 2 luteinizing hormone	12 u/L
Follicle-stimulating hormone	4 u/L
Prolactin	Normal
Sex hormone binding globulin	Reduced
Testosterone	High
Day 24 progesterone	4 nmol/L

Hysterosalpingogram demonstrates bilateral fill and spill of both tubes with a normal uterine cavity. The ultrasound scan of her ovaries is shown below.

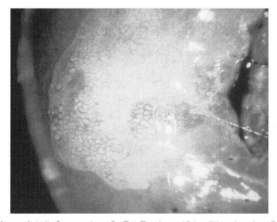

Figure 8.7   Reproduced from Monga A (ed) *Gynaecology By Ten Teachers*, 18th edition. London: Edward Arnold 2006.

a) What is the likely diagnosis?
b) How would you initially try to counsel and manage this patient?

11 Disorders of early pregnancy

A 17-year-old woman presents to the early pregnancy assessment unit complaining of 7 weeks' amenorrhoea, nausea and vomiting, breast tenderness, moderate bleeding and intermittent abdominal pain.

a) On examination, she has a normal pulse and blood pressure, there are no signs of peripheral shutdown, she has no adnexal tenderness, the cervix is closed and non-tender. Urinary pregnancy test is positive. What are the possible diagnoses?

b) A transvaginal scan demonstrates a gestation sac of 30 mm., a yolk sac, a fetal pole and a fetal heart is clearly seen beating. A large haematoma of 40 mm is seen adjacent to the gestation sac. A corpus luteum was noted on the right ovary measuring 25 mm and the left ovary was normal. There was no free fluid or any other adnexal mass noted. What are the diagnosis and your initial management?

c) Two weeks later, the woman returns for a repeat scan, as she has experienced further bleeding. On ultrasound, the gestation sac measures 29 mm, the yoke sac is seen but no fetal heart movements are seen. What would you do next?

12 Benign diseases of the uterus and cervix

a) Label this figure indicating the typical location of fibroids.

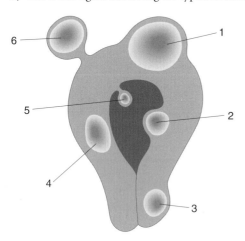

Figure 8.8 Adapted from Monga A (ed) *Gynaecology By Ten Teachers*, 18th edition. London: Edward Arnold 2006.

b) What are the typical clinical presentations of fibroids?
c) What are the different types of degeneration that fibroids can undergo?

13 Benign diseases of the uterus and cervix

A 34-year-old nulliparous woman from Ghana is referred by her general practitioner (GP) complaining of menorrhagia, dysmenorrhoea, urinary frequency, right loin pain and constipation. On examination, she is normotensive with a pulse of 98 beats per minute, she has pale sclerae and she has a pelvic mass, which is the same size as a 25-week pregnancy. Her last menstrual period was a week ago and was extremely heavy and has just stopped.

a) What are the possible diagnoses?
b) What investigations would you perform and why?
c) An ultrasound scan shows a large, fundal, subserous fibroid and several submucous fibroids, the largest being of 3 cm in diameter. They do not appear to impinge on the uterine cavity. The renal ultrasound scan shows normal renal tracts with no evidence of obstruction. A mid-stream urine confirms that the patient had a urinary tract infection; this was treated and her loin pain improved. Haemoglobin was low, with a mean corpuscular volume. What options would you offer to the patient?

14 Malignant diseases of the uterus and cervix

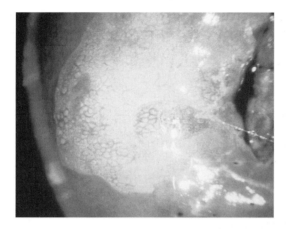

Figure 8.9   Courtesy of Mr KS Metcalf; reproduced from Monga A (ed) *Gynaecology By Ten Teachers*, 18th edition. London: Edward Arnold 2006.

a) What is shown in the picture above?
b) What does this colposcopic finding show?
c) What is the likely diagnosis?
d) What is the treatment for this condition?
e) Which virus strains are thought to be causative in developing this condition?
f) Why is it important to treat this?
g) What is the follow-up for these patients?

15 Infections in gynaecology

A 20-year-old woman presents with a 3-day history of pelvic pain, vaginal discharge and fever. She had unprotected intercourse 10 days ago with her new partner. On examination, she has cervical excitation, a mucopurulent discharge and tenderness in both adnexae.
a) What is the most likely diagnosis?
b) What is the commonest cause?
c) What are the other possible causes?
d) What cells do the main causative organisms colonize?
e) What tests are used to make the diagnosis?
f) What are the commonest treatments?
g) What other precautions have to be taken?
h) What are the risks associated with subsequent pregnancy?

16 Infections in gynaecology

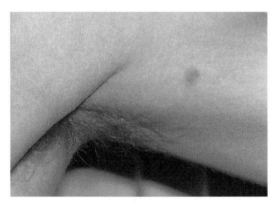

Figure 8.10   Reproduced from Monga A (ed) *Gynaecology By Ten Teachers*, 18th edition. London: Edward Arnold 2006.

a) What is seen in the photograph above?
b) What condition is this associated with and what is the causative organism?
c) What is the natural history of infection?
d) How is it transmitted?
e) What type of organism is the virus?
f) How does this replicate?
g) How is the diagnosis made and how is the disease monitored?
h) What is the treatment of choice?

17 Urogynaecology

This is a urinary diary of an 80-year-old woman who complains of urinary incontinence:

Time	Day 1		Day 2		Day 3	
	Volume in (mL)	Urine out (mL)	Volume in (mL)	Urine out (mL)	Volume in (mL)	Urine out (mL)
7 am		250		200		220
8 am	300		330		330	100
9 am		100		150		
10 am	200	75		100		100
11 am			330		200	50
12 pm		100		100		50
1 pm		100		75		
2 pm	175		200			100
3 pm		100		75	450	
4 pm		75		100		75
5 pm						50
6 pm	400	50	450	100		50
7 pm				50	450	
8 pm	100	100	330	50		100
9 pm	200	75		50		100
10 pm			330		300	
11 pm			100			100
12 am		100				

(*Continued*)

Time	Day 1		Day 2		Day 3	
	Volume in (mL)	Urine out (mL)	Volume in (mL)	Urine out (mL)	Volume in (mL)	Urine out (mL)
1 am				100		100
2 am		100				100
3 am		100		100		
4 am						100
5 am				100		
6 am						

a) What is this patient's bladder functional capacity?
b) What is the patient's daytime frequency?
c) What is the patient's night-time frequency?
d) What are the possible diagnoses?

The patient complains of leakage with coughing as well as urgency, frequency, nocturia and occasional urge incontinence. Formal cystometry is performed and the results are given below:

Maximum capacity	280 mL
First sensation	80 mL
First urgency	90 mL
Maximum detrusor pressure	A peak up to 20 cm of water was noted after a cough
Voided volume	320 mL
Flow rate	20 mL/second
Detrusor pressure at peak flow	60 cm of water

e) What is the diagnosis?
f) This woman had cystometry due to multiple mixed symptoms. What are the other indications for urodynamics?

18 Urogynaecology

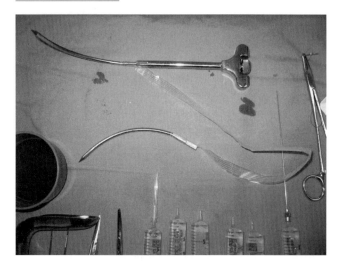

Figure 8.11

a) What does the picture above show?
b) What is it used to treat?
c) What was the traditional procedure used to treat USI?
d) What are the main consequences of colposuspension?
e) What are the advantages of TVT over colposuspension?

19 Uterovaginal prolapse

a) Label the diagram below.

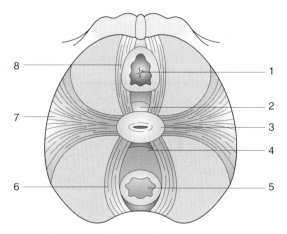

Figure 8.12   Reproduced from Lewis TLT, Chamberlain GVP (eds), *Gynaecology by Ten Teachers*, 15th edition. London: Edward Arnold 1990.

b) Describe the three mechanisms of support for pelvic organs.

20 Uterovaginal prolapse

Classification and grading of prolapse
a) Complete the following table:

Organ	Compartment	Nomenclature of prolapse
1	Anterior	7
2		8
3	Posterior	9
4		10
5	Apex	11
6		12

b) Describe the grading system with regards to primary, secondary and tertiary prolapse.

21 The menopause

A 50-year-old woman with no significant past obstetric history and no previous operations attends your clinic requesting hormone replacement therapy (HRT).
a) What are the contraindications to HRT?
b) What are the modes of delivery for HRT?
c) What are the sites of action of oestrogen?
d) When should progesterone be administered?
e) What are the two types of oestrogen and progesterone regime, and when should they be used?

22 Common gynaecological procedures

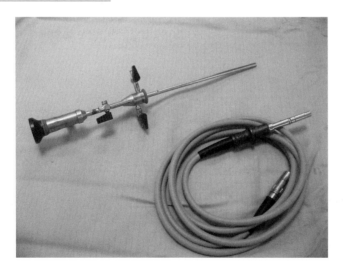

Figure 8.13

a) What is shown in this picture?
b) List indications for the use of this procedure.
c) List the complications of this procedure.

23 Common gynaecological procedures

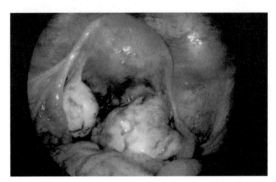

Figure 8.14 Reproduced from Monga A (ed) *Gynaecology By Ten Teachers*, 18th edition. London: Edward Arnold 2006.

a) What is the image seen in the photograph?
b) What is the instrument used to provide this image?
c) What are the indications for this procedure?
d) What are the complications of the procedure?

OSCE answers

1 History and examination

Name, age, occupation
Main presenting complaint
History of presenting complaint
- Menstrual history:
    - Pattern of bleeding (regular/irregular)
    - Amount of loss (clots/flooding/sanitary protection)
- Intermenstrual bleeding
- Pelvic pain: ? related to cycle, site and nature, radiation
- Dyspareunia (superficial/deep)
- Vaginal discharge
- Fertility history/urogynaecology questions

Menstrual cycle:
- Menarche
- Number of days bleeding/number of days between periods
- First day of last menstrual period

Past gynaecological history:
- Previous investigations and procedures
- Smear history

Past obstetric history:
- Number of previous pregnancies
- Number of previous live births, stillbirths, miscarriages, terminations
- Birth weights and mode of delivery of live births

Sexual and contraceptive history:
- Dyspareunia
- Sexually transmitted diseases
- Contraception

Previous medical history/drug history and allergies
Social history:
- Occupation
- Smoking and alcohol intake

Systemic enquiry

See Chapter 1, *Gynaecology by Ten Teachers*, 18th edition.

2 History and examination

Figure 8.1: Sims' speculum. The patient lies in the left lateral position; it is used to inspect the vault and anterior vaginal wall.

Figure 8.2: Cusco's (bivalve) speculum. The patient lies in the lithotomy position; it is used to inspect the exposed cervix.

See Chapter 1, *Gynaecology by Ten Teachers*, 18th edition.

3 Embryology, anatomy and physiology

Figure 8.3: 1, Right ureter; 2, ovary; 3, rectouterine fold; 4, posterior fornix; 5, cervix uteri; 6, rectal ampulla; 7, anal canal; 8, vagina; 9, urethra; 10, bladder; 11, vesicouterine recess; 12, fundus of uterus; 13, external iliac vessels; 14, ovarian ligament; 15, uterine tube; 16, suspensory ligament of ovary.

Figure 8.4: 1, Fundus; 2, peritoneum (serous layer); 3, oviduct; 4, myometrium; 5, endometrium; 6, anatomical internal os; 7, lateral fornix; 8, external os; 9, vagina; 10, cervix; 11, isthmus; 12, cornu; 13, body.

See Chapter 2, *Gynaecology by Ten Teachers*, 18th edition.

4 Normal and abnormal sexual development and puberty

a) Turner's syndrome.
b) 45XO.
c) Webbed neck, short stature, wide carrying angle of arms and widely spaced nipples.
d) Low levels of oestradiol with high levels of follicle-stimulating hormone (FSH) and luteinizing hormone (LH).
e) Macroscopically the ovaries appear streaked.
f) There are two phases of treatment. First, at puberty, hormone replacement therapy (HRT) is instigated for the development of secondary sexual characteristics. Second, when the patient wishes to become pregnant, she will require the aid of donor eggs and sperm, which could then be inserted into the uterus.

See Chapter 3, *Gynaecology by Ten Teachers*, 18th edition.

5 The normal menstrual cycle

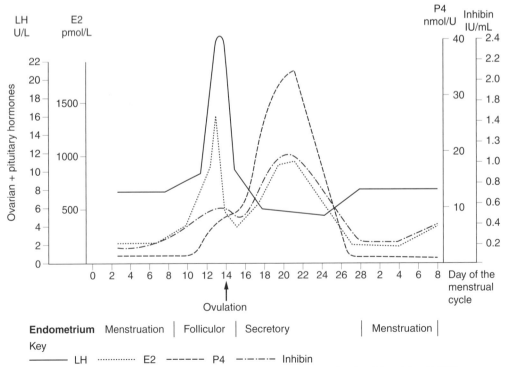

Figure 8.15 Adapted from Monga A (ed) *Gynaecology By Ten Teachers*, 18th edition. London: Edward Arnold 2006.

E2, oestradiol; LH, luteinizing hormone; P4, progesterone.

See Chapter 4, *Gynaecology by Ten Teachers*, 18th edition.

6 The normal menstrual cycle

Figure a	Figure b
Follicular phase	Luteal phase
Proliferative phase	Secretory phase
Glandular and stromal proliferation	Stromal oedema and glandular growth
Pre-ovulation	Postovulation
Oestrogen predominates	Progesterone predominates

See Chapter 4, *Gynaecology by Ten Teachers*, 18th edition.

7 Fertility control

Contraceptive method	Failure rate per 100 women years
Combined oral contraceptive pill	0.1–1
Progesterone-only pill	1–3
Depo-Provera	0.1–2
Implanon	0
Copper-bearing intrauterine device (IUD)	1–2
Levonorgestrel-releasing IUD	0.5
Male condom	2–5
Female diaphragm	1–15
Persona	6
Natural family planning	2–3
Vasectomy	0.02
Female sterilization	0.13

See Chapter 6, *Gynaecology by Ten Teachers*, 18th edition.

8 Fertility control

Patients who have forgotten to take their pill should be counselled using the following algorithm.

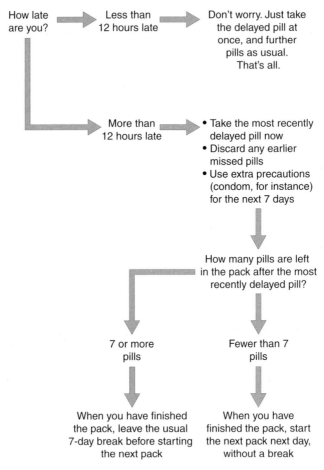

Figure 8.16 Reproduced with permission from Loudon N, Glasier A, Gebbie A (eds), *Handbook of family planning and reproductive health care*, 3rd edn. London: Churchill Livingstone 2000.

See Chapter 6, *Gynaecology by Ten Teachers*, 18th edition.

9 Fertility control

Contraceptive method	Inhibition of ovulation	Barrier between gametes	Effect on cervical mucus and prevention of implantation	Toxicity to male gametes
Combined oral contraceptive pill	+	−	+	−
Progesterone-only pill	4%	−	+	−
Depo	+	−	+	−
IUD	−	−	+	+
IUS	−	−	+	−
Condoms	−	+	−	−
Natural family planning	−	+	−	−
Female sterilization	−	+	−	−
Male sterilization	−	+	−	−

See Chapter 6, *Gynaecology by Ten Teachers*, 18th edition.

10 Infertility

a) Polycystic ovary syndrome.

b) One should initially counsel the patient regarding the diagnosis and implications of polycystic ovary syndrome. Explain that polycystic ovary syndrome is a condition typified by insulin resistance, an irregular cycle, hirsutism and weight gain. The main problems are anovulation, irregular periods and women usually present either because of oligomenorrhoea and wanting a regular cycle (these women are usually treated with the combined oral contraceptive pill) or infertility. One should also explain that there are risks of unopposed oestrogen and that there is a slightly higher risk of endometrial carcinoma later on in life if these patients do not have progesterone. There is also a risk of developing hypercholesterolaemia and non-insulin-dependent diabetes mellitus in later life.

If patients reduce their body mass index by 5 per cent, 30 per cent will achieve ovulation spontaneously and those that do not will be much more receptive to ovulation induction. Ovulation induction can be in the form of oral clomifene citrate or by gonadotrophin therapy, if patients are clomifene resistant. It is important to discuss the risks of multiple pregnancy and ovarian hyperstimulation, if ovulation induction is embarked upon.

See Chapter 7, *Gynaecology by Ten Teachers*, 18th edition.

11 Disorders of early pregnancy

a) A threatened miscarriage with a viable intrauterine pregnancy, a non-viable intrauterine pregnancy (missed miscarriage/incomplete miscarriage), ectopic pregnancy and molar pregnancy.

b) The diagnosis is a threatened miscarriage with a viable intrauterine pregnancy. Initially, one should reassure the mother that the fetus is viable and the fetal heart can be seen. One should explain the presence of the haematoma has demonstrated some bleeding. It may resolve but she may have further bleeding and may still lose the pregnancy. Initially, one would plan to rescan the pregnancy in 2 weeks' time to confirm viability and see if the haematoma is resolving. However, you should explain to the patient that she may have further bleeding/pain, which may suggest that she is miscarrying, and if this does occur, she should return to the hospital. She should be given a telephone number to contact the hospital at all times.

c) Explain to the patient that the pregnancy is now not viable and that she will need to have the uterus evacuated. This can be done either by expectant, medical or surgical procedures. Surgical evacuation is the most effective, but those managed with expectant and medical management are efficient in 50 and 65 per cent of cases, respectively. One should give the woman contact numbers for self-help groups, for support groups and also a contact number, if she wishes any further information. She should be given advice about subsequent pregnancies and that usually one would advise her to refrain from trying to conceive again until she has had subsequent periods.

See Chapter 8, *Gynaecology by Ten Teachers*, 18th edition.

12 Benign diseases of the uterus and cervix

a) 1, Subserous; 2, submucosal; 3, cervical; 4, intramural; 5, intracavity polyp; 6, pedunculated fibroid.
b) Menorrhagia, pelvic mass, pressure symptoms (urinary frequency), pain (if fibroid is undergoing degeneration).
c) Red, hyaline, cystic, calcification, malignant.

See Chapter 9, *Gynaecology by Ten Teachers*, 18th edition.

13 Benign diseases of the uterus and cervix

a) The most likely diagnoses is fibroids, but an ovarian cyst with concomitant menorrhagia and adenomyosis is also possible. It is likely that the pelvic mass is causing related pressure symptoms, with urinary frequency resulting from pressure against the bladder and possible right ureteric compression by the fibroid causing renal dilatation.
b) The following investigations would be performed.
   • A full blood count to exclude anaemia.
   • A pelvic ultrasound scan to determine the nature of the mass to try to distinguish a fibroid from an ovarian mass.
   • A computerized tomography scan may be necessary, if there are inconclusive results from the ultrasound scan.
   • A renal ultrasound scan/intravenous pyelogram to assess whether there is ureteric obstruction and dilatation of the renal pelvices.
   • Hysteroscopy may be necessary to assess the uterine cavity.
c) As the patient is relatively asymptomatic from her anaemia, she could have iron supplementation rather than risk a blood transfusion. Depending on her fertility wishes, one would need to discuss the following treatments.
   • Mirena, if her uterine cavity is normal; this may give some symptomatic relief.
   • Transcervical resection of the fibroid, if the main problem is from the submucous fibroid.
   • A myomectomy, if the patient wishes to retain fertility.
   • Total abdominal hysterectomy, the patient does not wish to remain fertile.
   • Selective angiographic embolization is a new treatment for fibroids but cannot be used if a woman wants to become pregnant in the future.
   • It is always worth giving adjunctive gonadotrophin-releasing hormone agonist pre-treatment for 2–3 months to reduce the bulk of vascularity of fibroids prior to surgery.

See Chapter 9, *Gynaecology by Ten Teachers*, 18th edition.

14 Malignant diseases of the uterus and cervix

a) Colposcopy of the cervix.

b) Acetowhite staining, mosaicism and punctuation.

c) Cervical intraepithelial neoplasia 3.

d) Large loop excision of the transformation zone (LLETZ).

e) Human papillomavirus (HPV) strains 16 and 18 are the most commonly associated with cervical cancer.

f) Cervical intraepithelial neoplasia (CIN) has the potential to develop to an invasive malignancy, although in itself does not have malignant properties. Treatment, therefore, involves removing the abnormal cells completely down to a depth of 10 mm.

g) Current guidelines recommend a smear and colposcopy at 6 months after the large loop excision of the transformation zone (LLETZ) procedure, then a smear by the GP 12 months post-LLETZ and then annually for 9 years. After this, if the smears remain normal, the patient can go back to having 3-yearly smears.

See Chapter 12, *Gynaecology by Ten Teachers*, 18th edition.

15 Infections in gynaecology

a) Acute pelvic inflammatory disease.

b) Chlamydia.

c) Ascending infection from instrumentation of the uterus/intrauterine contraceptive device (IUCD) usage, previous pelvic surgery, appendicitis, sexually transmitted diseases, such as gonorrhoea.

d) The columnar cells of the cervix.

e) ELISA (enzyme-linked immunosorbent assay). This is the commonest investigation; however, it has limited sensitivity. Direct fluorescent antibody test (DFA) can be performed, which is more specific.

f) Doxycycline and azithromycin.

g) Contact tracing and treatment of other sexual partners.

h) Ectopic pregnancy.

See Chapter 15, *Gynaecology by Ten Teachers*, 18th edition.

16 Infections in gynaecology

a) Kaposi's sarcoma.

b) The condition is the acquired immunodeficiency syndrome (AIDS), which is caused by the human immunodeficiency virus (HIV).

c) 20 per cent of people who acquire HIV have an acute seroconversion illness typified by fever, generalized lymphadenopathy and a maculate erythematous rash, pharyngitis and conjunctivitis. The majority of people are asymptomatic. Affected individuals then develop a steady decline in their immune function over a number of years. This usually presents with non-life-threatening opportunistic infections, such as recurrent candidiasis, shingles and frequent episodes of genital or oral herpes. Hairy oral leukoplakia may come and go, and is pathopneumonic of immunodeficiency. If left untreated, full-blown AIDS will develop usually within 10 years.

d) Transmission is by sexual intercourse and contamination with blood products, such as needle stick injury.

e) It is a single-stranded RNA retrovirus.

f) The gp120 protein binds to the CD4 receptor of the T cells. It then hijacks the cell and uses the viral reverse transcriptase enzyme to produce viral DNA.

g) Seroconversion can be determined by finding antibodies to the gp120 protein. The disease is monitored by measuring the CD4 lymphocyte count.

h) Combination antiviral drugs are used, which target the reverse transcriptase enzyme and viral proteases. These do improve life expectancy but are expensive.

See Chapter 15, *Gynaecology by Ten Teachers*, 18th edition.

17 Urogynaecology

a) 100 mL.
b) 10–11.
c) 3.
d) Detrusor overactivity or urinary tract infection.
e) The likely diagnosis is detrusor overactivity. This is due to the fact that a rise in detrusor pressure was seen on filling. In addition, the patient complained of urgency in association with a rise in detrusor pressure and this confirmed detrusor overactivity.
f) Previous unsuccessful continence surgery, voiding disorder, neuropathic bladder, investigation prior to embarking on incontinence surgery.

See Chapter 16, *Gynaecology by Ten Teachers*, 18th edition.

18 Urogynaecology

a) Tension-free vaginal tape (TVT) sling.
b) Urodynamic-proven stress incontinence (USI).
c) Colposuspension.
d) 70–90 per cent long-term success in treating stress incontinence. Long-term risk of poor voiding (5 per cent), *de novo* detrusor overactivity (5 per cent), intermittent self-catheterization ($<$ 1 per cent) and rectocele.
e) Performed under local anaesthetic, less invasive, shorter hospital stay, quicker recovery, similar success rates but less risk of voiding disorder, *de novo* detrusor overactivity and no increased risk of developing a rectocele.

See Chapter 16, *Gynaecology by Ten Teachers*, 18th edition.

19 Uterovaginal prolapse

a) 1, Internal urethral orifice; 2, vagina; 3, cervix; 4, rectovaginal pouch; 5, rectum; 6, uterosacral ligament; 7, transverse cervical (cardinal) ligament; 8, pubocervical fascia.
b) The mechanisms of support for pelvic organs are:
   • Muscular supports of the levator ani which forms the pelvic diaphragm.
   • Endofascial supports in the form of the uterosacral, cardinal and pubocervical ligaments.
   • The posterior angulation of the vagina, thus preventing pelvic organs falling through the vagina when the patient is standing.

See Chapter 17, *Gynaecology by Ten Teachers*, 18th edition.

20 Uterovaginal prolapse

a) 1, Urethra; 2, bladder; 3, rectum; 4, omentum/small bowel; 5, uterus; 6, vault; 7, urethrocele; 8, cystocele; 9, rectocele; 10, enterocele; 11, uterine prolapse; 12, vault prolapse.
b) Grading:
   • Primary prolapse is deviation from its anatomical position but not to the level of the hymenal ring/introitus.
   • Secondary prolapse is deviation of the organ from its anatomical position to the level of the introitus but not beyond.
   • Tertiary prolapse is deviation of the organ from its anatomical position beyond the hymenal ring.

See Chapter 17, *Gynaecology by Ten Teachers*, 18th edition.

21 The menopause

a) Absolute contraindications include present or suspected pregnancy, suspicion of breast cancer, suspicion of endometrial cancer, acute active liver disease, uncontrolled hypertension or confirmed venous thrombotic event. Relative contraindications include the presence of uterine fibroids, a past history of benign breast disease, unconfirmed venous thromboembolic episode, chronic stable liver disease and migraine.

b) Topical, oral, transdermal and subcutaneous implant.

c) Bone (arrests and reverses bone loss), cardiovascular system (reduces vasomotor symptoms, alters lipid profile and increases risk of venous thrombosis), genitourinary system (reduces atrophy) and central nervous system.

d) Progesterone is required to protect the endometrium in women who have not had a hysterectomy.

e) Sequential HRT for women below 54 or who have been amenorrhoeic for less than 2 years, and continuous combined HRT for women over 54 who have been amenorrhoeic for <2 years.

See Chapter 18, *Gynaecology by Ten Teachers*, 18th edition.

22 Common gynaecological procedures

a) Rigid hysteroscope.

b) Postmenopausal bleeding, irregular menstruation/intermenstrual bleeding in women over the age of 35, persistent menorrhagia, persistent discharge, suspected uterine malformation and suspected Asherman's syndrome.

c) Complications include perforation of the uterus and cervical damage at the time of cervical dilatation, risk of infection and ascending of infection, if already present.

See Appendix 1, *Gynaecology by Ten Teachers*, 18th edition.

23 Common gynaecological procedures

a) This is a laparoscopic view of endometriosis. Endometriosis is scored using the American fertility scoring system.

b) The instrument is called a laparoscope.

c) The indications for laparoscopy include suspected ectopic pregnancy, undiagnosed pelvic pain, tubal patency testing, and sterilization or an operative laparoscopy.

d) Complications include damage to intra-abdominal structures, such as the bowel or major blood vessels. Herniation through port sites is also possible through larger port sites, such as a 10 mm or larger port.

See Appendix 1 and 2, *Gynaecology by Ten Teachers*, 18th edition.

Index